What Therapists Need to Know About Perinatal and Early Relational Health

What Therapists Need to Know About Perinatal and Early Relational Health is a vital and timely text that will strengthen any clinician's awareness and competence when working with children, infants, and caregivers. All the chapters are written from a framework of cultural humility to support the competent care of individuals with different intersectionalities. Cultural humility involves critical self-reflection and critique of values, beliefs, and experiences, and so each chapter provides reflective questions and tools that support clinicians' anti-oppressive practices.

What Therapists Need to Know About Perinatal and Early Relational Health offers practical strategies that are rooted in diversity-informed tenets and support reflection on our values, beliefs, and experiences. By embracing the wisdom within these pages, therapists can transform their practice into one that is more relational and heart-centered.

Meyleen Velasquez, DSW, LICSW, RPT-S™, PMH-C, IMH-E®, is an immigrant Latina psychotherapist specializing in perinatal and infant mental health through an anti-oppressive framework.

What Therapists Need to Know About Perinatal and Early Relational Health

A Guide to Anti-Oppressive Counseling with Caregivers, Babies, and Young Children

Meyleen M. Velasquez

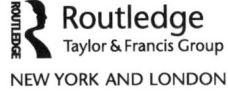

Routledge
Taylor & Francis Group
NEW YORK AND LONDON

Designed cover image: eclipse images © Getty Images

First published 2025
by Routledge
605 Third Avenue, New York, NY 10158

and by Routledge
4 Park Square, Milton Park, Abingdon, Oxon, OX14 4RN

Routledge is an imprint of the Taylor & Francis Group, an informa business

ISBN: 978-1-032-25652-8 (hbk)
ISBN: 978-1-032-25650-4 (pbk)
ISBN: 978-1-003-28639-4 (ebk)

DOI: 10.4324/9781003286394

Typeset in Helvetica
by SPi Technologies India Pvt Ltd (Straive)

For you, for me, for all of us. May it be of benefit.

Contents

Figures

Acknowledgments

My heart is full when I think of all who came before me, those here with me, and those who will come after me with a heart to support babies, young children, and their families. We are together in this cycle.

A special shout-out goes to Dr. Megan Covington from The People's Editor, whose content editing, anti-racist frame, and direct feedback supported my whole soul while writing this text. Please check her company out!

I am grateful to the Tenets Initiative and the Irving Harris Foundation for allowing me to reprint the "Diversity-informed tenets for work with infants, children & families" in this text. I also thank Perinatal Support Washington for allowing me to reproduce their Wellness Plan.

I also want to acknowledge Dr. Karen Slovak, my incredible mentor during my doctoral journey. Thank you for your feedback and responsiveness. You are a gem in academia.

To my dear husband, I acknowledge you for giving me an example of a loving relationship and the experience of being seen and heard.

About the Author

Meyleen Velasquez, DSW, LICSW, RPT-S™, PMH-C, IMH-E®, is an immigrant Latina psychotherapist specializing in perinatal and infant mental health. Meyleen has a doctorate in social work and focused her research on anti-racist and anti-oppressive mental health services. Her practice supports birthing people and clinicians working from an anti-oppressive framework. Meyleen identified as a Brown person for most of her life until several years ago when Vitiligo changed how she navigates the world.

She sits on the Alliance for the Advancement of Infant Mental Health's board. Meyleen has served as a board member for the Washington Association for Infant Mental Health, Chair for the Florida Chapter of Postpartum Support International, and the past President of the Florida Association for Play Therapy. She enjoys training, speaking, and writing and believes the more we can support each other, the better for our communities. You can follow her on YouTube or Instagram @meyleenvelasquez or at www.hummingbirdcounseling.com.

Introduction

CHAPTER ONE

Bridging the Gaps Observed
Reflections on Counseling Perinatal Caregivers and Their Little Ones

May our hearts help us light up our world.

This book proposes a decolonized, anti-oppressive model for supporting pregnant individuals and families with young children. I aim to support you in creating a bridge between infant, perinatal, and play therapy so that families can be seen and heard in their fullness. Relationships are the cornerstone of our communities. In genuine relationships, we are seen and heard. As I see myself reflected in you, I can connect with my strength and push on. Sometimes, the only way I can push forward is by being with someone who can help me see my strength. To be *with* means to have your whole-self honored. It means that no part of you is unwelcomed. All that you are, have experienced, survived, and celebrated makes you who you are: unique, extraordinary, and unforgettable. I hope this sacred truth grounds you to yourself, your clinical work, and those whom you love and support. Our capacity to connect with who we are promotes healing. It is a message that I hope you can share with the individuals, children, and families you support. Divisiveness is one of the many impacts of colonization in our field. Clinicians desiring to work with caregivers and babies must generally choose between working with the adult, the child, or the dyadic relationship. This division often creates added barriers for caregivers in need of supportive services. As I conceptualized this text, I wanted readers to think with me about relational work, systemic racism, and supporting families with babies and young children. There is a part of me that feels nervous about challenging ways of treatment and also presenting information that you may already know. However, I learned we must push through that fear and speak our truth. I wonder if this way of being can support us in grounding deeply in ourselves. I am inviting you into a journey of ambiguity and questioning ways of being and practicing. I hope you will accept this

DOI: 10.4324/9781003286394-2

invitation and extend it to the families you support. This chapter explores my journey as a human social worker and the gaps in cross-training I observed while working with perinatal individuals, children, and clinicians.

THE JOURNEY

I came into the mental health field with a heart full of hope and a desire to leave the world a little better than I found it. I dreamed of working with a population where I could significantly impact my community. Like many mental health providers, my education involved a Bachelor's and a Master's degree. I trained in play therapy, infant and early childhood mental health (IECMH), and eventually, in working with pregnant and postpartum people. Much of my training focused on the individual actions I could take with clients to impact their well-being. Play therapy was my first advanced training. It taught me how to interpret a child's world and to support emotional healing using toys as our language. I learned the magic of expressive skills like singing, painting, playing, and creating stories. This way of practicing felt attuned to how my ancestors navigated the world. Play therapy connects with me as no other set of skills does. Play is a way of being. In my continued search for where I could be the most helpful, I found a whole world of supporting babies and young children. The early relational field, known by its more official names of IECMH and infant mental health (IMH), is a discipline like no other. It is reflective, relational, and attuned to the needs of a child and the relationship with their caregiver. Most of the work done by early relationship specialists involves using toys and conversations with caregivers. The caregiver engagement in working with babies marked my interest in building a bridge to be relational and attuned to the specific needs of all the individuals involved when I worked with families.

The more I worked with babies and young children, the more I noticed aspects of the caregivers' identity that went overlooked. My work involved supporting adults in being safe, protective, and reliable caregivers to their children. This goal is vital, as babies and toddlers are one of the most vulnerable populations. Babies cannot protect themselves when others hurt them. However, I noted that the parent's identity in the counseling relationship was rooted in their capacity to meet their child's needs. While this role is crucial, as little ones depend entirely on the people around them, it leaves the caregiver's *individualhood* out of the picture. A person who becomes a parent loses their identity as an individual almost from the moment of pregnancy. They receive unsolicited advice from everyone, including strangers, about caring for their pregnancy. They might lose their name as others refer to them as "mom," "dad," "baba," and so on, which, although cute, might feel like the beginning of chipping away at the self. The part of ourselves that holds individualhood does not automatically disappear when someone becomes a caregiver. It remains ever-present and hungry to be recognized. The longer it goes unseen, the worse an individual might feel.

I wondered what was missing in the treatment and interventions I provided. I wanted more for myself and for the people I served. A series of Google searches led me to a training on perinatal mood and anxiety disorders. The perinatal period is the time between pregnancy and up to two years after delivery or post-partum. Would it be dramatic to say that the training changed my life? It did change a part of me. It lit a bulb in my mind and showed me a whole way of supporting families that seemed so evident while so forgotten: the parent as a person with needs and desires distinct from their caregiver role. We know this idea is accurate, yet it can be hard to hold the competing demands of the care-giver and their children in counseling. One of the reasons the bridge between the fields is challenging is that most master-level programs do not offer specific training on assessing and treating perinatal populations, babies, or young chil-dren. Post-graduation, we find that most advanced clinical training programs separate the mental health needs of adults and children. Our humanity is not binary. The well-being of a system does not rest on the "health" of one part without attention to everything else. The field of mental health is a construct of colonization. It is filled with divisions and hierarchies.

What we know to be true is that people healed in communities well before the onset of Western psychology in the 1800s (Menjivar, 2022). The separation of play, infant, and perinatal fields is how clinicians have worked within a domi-nant, colonial lens. We can practice differently. We can honor the interconnect-edness of humans to each other and to the earth. We can also support the notion that we are individuals and part of a whole. The part of us connected to the *whole* needs attention as much if not many more times than the others.

ON SOCIAL POSITIONING

Before continuing, I would like to engage in critical practices to ground this work in an anti-colonialist approach. I begin this section with a land acknowledgment. I want to acknowledge that I am a settler on the stolen land of the Coast Salish peoples. The first people of Seattle are the Duwamish. I was born in Venezuela, in the land of the Timotes people, and grew up in the land of the Arawakos people. I invite readers to join me in honoring the Coast Salish, Timotes, and Arawakos peoples and their protection of the land, elders, and future genera-tions. I encourage you to think about whose land you inhabit and came from and take time to learn and honor the Indigenous communities who have been here since time immemorial.

Acknowledging whose land we are in is a move towards recognition of Indigenous people and a step towards resisting the erasure of history. A land acknowledgment becomes meaningful when we take steps to learn about the history and local treaties (and ways they were violated) and take action to support Indigenous communities (Native Governance Center, 2021). Please take time to think about what action will look like for you. I will share some steps I take to remain accountable here. Note that these are not aspirational in any way. Instead, it is a way for me to show my humanity and areas for growth and to reflect on settlerhood out loud.

- I make a monthly donation to the Duwamish Tribe. You can learn about voluntary land taxes in your area if you are interested in doing this.
- I am learning about the history and current context of Indigenous communities in my state, where I was born, and where I grew up.
- I aspire to intentionally name Indigenous communities when speaking and writing about the mental health field.

It is vital to identify who we are whenever we enter anti-oppressive spaces. I can share that I am a social worker in private practice with a love for working with babies, young children, and birthing people. I can go into detail about the letters behind my name, but that does not give you a felt experience of who I am as a human. I am a multiethnic Latina immigrant living in the U.S.A. I am the daughter of immigrants. My maternal family is Cuban, and my paternal family is Colombian. I grew up with my maternal family, who were forced to leave Cuba and settle in Venezuela following the revolution. The impact of imperialism also forced us to relocate to the U.S.A. in the mid-1990s. I am learning to hold my identity as a settler in the U.S.A. and someone whose land and people were and are deeply impacted by colonization. I am a formerly undocumented individual who grew up in poverty and survived trauma. I am neurodivergent, middle class, a U.S. citizen, cisgender, and married to a man. I am also a Brown woman navigating the world with Vitiligo. I spent much of my life trying to beat my body into submission by keeping it small before realizing I was trying to erase my Latinidad (Latin American identity). I wanted to meet a standard of beauty that is entirely made up and harms all. My life experiences guide my work, how I sit with people, and how I think about relationships. We can increase awareness of biases by reflecting on our culture and history. Turning the eye inward is the starting point for reflective practice. This practice can support clinicians in bringing their whole-selves into the counseling relationship and, hopefully, creating space to welcome the entire self of the people we support. I invite you to pause here and reflect on your identities.

In this work, I want to bring an anti-racist and anti-oppressive framework to the forefront of how we work with families. Kendi (2019) explained, "Anti-racism is a powerful collection of antiracist policies that lead to racial equity and are substantiated by antiracist ideas" (p. 20). Anti-racist policies and ideas aim to reach or maintain equity among racial groups. For instance, Black birthing people are 53 times more likely to die in childbirth than their White counterparts (American Society of Anesthesiologists, 2022). Anti-racist policies at the macro-level establish systems to collect data on racial disparities and implement community-driven steps such as access to doula care to address gaps (Opoku-Agyeman, 2022). In therapy with families and young children, anti-racism means active work to remove practices that benefit one racial group over another. One of the steps we take in a clinical program I co-manage at Perinatal Support Washington is thinking about access to services. We provide all services via telehealth. While this format was due to the pandemic, it allows us to serve clients across the state, including individuals in rural areas and those who might not have transportation. We also partner with clients and clinicians to think about the technology gap and develop creative ways to access services for those without internet access or low technological comfort. For instance, we might mail intake paperwork to someone unable to navigate our electronic health record platform or offer text-messaging support to someone who cannot participate in a talk therapy session. A provider striving to be anti-racist acknowledges the ways that racism impacts the lives of Black and Brown communities and actively works to integrate a reparative lens into clinical services (Cénat, 2020). Repairing entails taking action that promotes healing and liberation. Racism upholds structures that sustain oppression. Anti-oppressive practices call for a shift in balancing hierarchies of power dynamics between groups. We create space to honor the other when we deeply ground who we are. Check out Chapter 2 for the theoretical framework for this text.

THE HEART

The heart of this work resides in relationships. Authentic and attuned connections that aim to liberate all involved are the heart and soul of this work for me. Liberation in our clinical work entails active client participation in all aspects of care (Montero & Sonn, 2009). This lens focuses on removing barriers that harm and marginalize communities. The tricky thing about removing obstacles is that they are often invisible when we do not experience them. Barriers come in many forms. They include access to treatment and, many times, the treatment itself. Recently, I was hit with the reality that I am an expert in Westernized, dominant, and colonized ways of being. I did not like it, as you can imagine. However, moving towards anti-oppression entails sitting with discomfort. BIPOC people and individuals with intersecting marginalized identities are constantly uncomfortable. Taking an intentional turn with discomfort is vital for growth. As you move through your practice and learn new skills, I encourage you to think about the following three questions:

- Who developed this intervention/tool/practice?
- Who was it designed for?
- Whom was it tested on?

By answering these questions, we usually find the harmful historical and present-day lack of representation of people from the global majority and individuals with other marginalized identities. This lack of representation is a legacy of colonization and chattel slavery, which we can understand as structural racism. Research leads to funding and the implementation of interventions. However, when the studies center on something different than lived experience, interventions miss the culturally specific needs of the populations they aim to support. As I mentioned, the good news is that people have been healing in their communities since time immemorial. When we can move away from the idea of the therapist as the expert and knowledge holder, we can rely on communities' wisdom to guide healing and liberation.

I want to acknowledge that as much as I am looking to break free from harmful discourses, they are still present in everything I do. Racism, oppression, and white supremacy are the ocean we all swim in. They are at the center of all policies and interventions. Racism and oppression determine how we see each other. They form the automatic thoughts that judge a person of color before they have a chance to speak. These automatic thoughts result in asking someone, "Where are you from?" when whiteness is not detected or assuming that a person of color caring for a lighter-skinned child is the nanny. Those of us who hold non-Black and non-Indigenous identities must stay vigilant of how oppression and racism are present in our lives and work. Promoting liberation and justice means we agree to make the unknown known and the unseen visible. The unknown includes learning from individuals with lived experience and practicing self-awareness. The unseen can consist of addressing barriers that communities face, covert racism, and harmful organizational policies that further marginalize communities. If we go back to the metaphor of the heart, we can say that as long as we strive towards justice, the heart is beating. Oxygen flows as we learn and take action. The moment we stop reflecting and taking social justice-based action, relationships die. I encourage you to hold the words in this book with a sense of critical reflection, knowing there is no right way to practice or any perfectly anti-oppressive guide to meet everyone's diverse needs. I offer my experience in hopes that families will benefit, and you will be inspired to continue your anti-oppressive journey.

THE TENETS

As a part of modeling anti-oppression, I want to introduce an existing resource to help clinicians guide the heart of this work. "The diversity-informed tenets for work with children, infants and families" (Tenets) is a guide to anti-oppression. You can review the Tenets below. The Tenets were developed in 2011 by a diverse group of IECMH professionals organized in a workgroup by the Irving Harris Foundation. The Tenets "are a set of ten strategies and tools for strengthening the commitment and capacity of professionals, organizations, and systems that serve infants, children and families to embed diversity, inclusion and equity principles into their work" (Tenets Initiative, 2018, para. 1). The ten principles guide providers and systems to actively examine oppression and combat discrimination in their work with children and families. The work starts with a focus on self-awareness. Attempts at support not grounded in individual reflection and critique of power, privilege, discrimination, and racism lead to services perpetuating harm. Each Tenet is an aspiration goal moving us to examine how we work and partner with communities individually and systemically. I will highlight areas in this book where the Tenets come up as a way to utilize a highly valuable tool available for all. If you want to learn more about the Tenets and acquire official training, please visit https://diversityinformedtenets.org.

DIVERSITY-INFORMED TENETS FOR WORK WITH INFANTS, CHILDREN, AND FAMILIES

Irving Harris Foundation Professional Development Network Tenets Working Group

CENTRAL PRINCIPLE FOR DIVERSITY-INFORMED PRACTICE

Self-Awareness Leads to Better Services for Families: Working with infants, children, and families requires all individuals, organizations, and systems of care to reflect on our own culture, values, and beliefs, and on the impact that racism, classism, sexism, able-ism, homophobia, xenophobia, and other systems of oppression have had on our lives in order to provide diversity-informed, culturally attuned services.

STANCE TOWARDS INFANTS, CHILDREN, AND FAMILIES FOR DIVERSITY-INFORMED PRACTICE

Champion Children's Rights Globally: Infants and children are citizens of the world. The global community is responsible for supporting parents/caregivers, families, and local communities in welcoming, protecting, and nurturing them.

Work to Acknowledge Privilege and Combat Discrimination: Discriminatory policies and practices that harm adults harm the infants and children in their care. Privilege constitutes injustice. Diversity-informed practitioners acknowledge privilege where we hold it, and use it strategically and responsibly. We combat racism, classism, sexism, able-ism, homophobia, xenophobia, and other systems of oppression within ourselves, our practices, and our fields.

Recognize and Respect Non-Dominant Bodies of Knowledge: Diversity-informed practice recognizes non-dominant ways of knowing, bodies of knowledge, sources of strength, and routes to healing within all families and communities.

Honor Diverse Family Structures: Families decide who is included and how they are structured; no particular family constellation or organization is inherently optimal compared to any other. Diversity-informed practice recognizes and strives to counter the historical bias towards idealizing (and conversely blaming) biological mothers while overlooking the critical childrearing contributions of other parents and caregivers including second mothers, fathers, kin and felt family, adoptive parents, foster parents, and early care and educational providers.

PRINCIPLES FOR DIVERSITY-INFORMED RESOURCE ALLOCATION

Understand That Language Can Hurt or Heal: Diversity-informed practice recognizes the power of language to divide or connect, denigrate or celebrate, hurt or heal. We strive to use language (including body language, imagery, and other modes of nonverbal communication) in ways that most inclusively support all children and their families, caregivers, and communities.

Support Families in Their Preferred Language: Families are best supported in facilitating infants' and children's development and mental health when services are available in their native languages.

Allocate Resources to Systems Change: Diversity and inclusion must be proactively considered when doing any work with or on behalf of infants, children, and families. Resource allocation includes time, money, additional/alternative practices, and other supports and accommodations, otherwise systems of oppression may be inadvertently reproduced. Individuals, organizations, and systems of care need ongoing opportunities for reflection in order to identify implicit bias, remove barriers, and work to dismantle the root causes of disparity and inequity.

Make Space and Open Pathways: Infant, child, and family-serving workforces are most dynamic and effective when historically and currently marginalized individuals and groups have equitable access to a wide range of roles, disciplines, and modes of practice and influence.

ADVOCACY TOWARDS DIVERSITY, INCLUSION, AND EQUITY IN INSTITUTIONS

Advance Policy That Supports All Families: Diversity-informed practitioners consider the impact of policy and legislation on all people and advance a just and equitable policy agenda for and with families.

Diversity is used in the most inclusive sense possible, signaling race and ethnicity, as well as other identity markers, and referring to groups and individuals on both the "up and down side of power" along all axes.

Diversity-informed practice is a dynamic system of beliefs and values that strives for the highest levels of diversity, inclusion, and equity. Diversity-informed practice recognizes the historic and contemporary systems of oppression that shape interactions between individuals, organizations, and systems of care. Diversity-informed practice seeks the highest possible standard of equity, inclusivity, and justice in all spheres of practice: teaching and training, research and writing, public policy and advocacy and direct service.

The Tenets were collaboratively generated by a Working Group of the Harris Professional Development Network. They are reproduced with permission from the Tenets Initiative and the Irving Harris Foundation (© 2012 by the Irving Harris Foundation).

THE GAP

Building an authentic relationship requires our full self and allowing the other person(s) to bring their fullness into a co-created space. As we sit with clients in counseling, we bring who we are, including identities and experiences, as they are present, whether we share them or not. The same is true for the client. The fullness of who they are and what they have experienced is always present. As we think about creating clinical relationships, we must consider how we are co-creating ways that honor the fullness of the other to be seen and heard. Being seen and heard happens when sharing our story with someone who can hold all the parts. Our advanced clinical training might have focused on one specific population or a modality within a particular age group. For example, most Eye Movement Desensitization and Reprocessing (EMDR) basic training focuses on working with adults. Training in a play therapy model with clients aged 3 and over may not include how to support the caregiver through a perinatal complication. Similarly, perinatal training can easily miss crucial signs of developmental or relational concerns for the baby. IECMH therapists generally focus on the caregiver–child relationship and may miss some of the birthing person's perinatal mental health (PMH) complications. If a therapist notices an emotional concern, they might provide a referral for outside support.

Making a referral for a complementary provider is an appropriate and common practice. For some families, external support might be accessible regarding their availability to make and attend an appointment, financial capacity for payment or co-payment, and emotional bandwidth. For many others, the thought of meeting another provider is daunting. Many families I have supported throughout the years do not immediately jump at the idea of an additional provider. Even when financial resources are available, families are busy. We live in a culture that does not support families, so the demands of work and life are exhausting. It is hard having to re-tell our story to multiple people, not knowing if they will be the right person for you. It is also hard to find a therapist online, only to find out that they are unavailable. Let us layer into that example the experiences of a family holding multiple marginalized identities. The emotional bandwidth required to make phone calls and organize appointments might take a higher toll on them/us. These experiences chip away at our emotional bandwidth.

I am sitting with a two-fold reality: clinicians need high-quality, advanced training, *and* families are suffering in silence right now. Suffering does not wait to strike until there is a provider available or one who has the "right" training. Unfortunately, suffering and distress are the here-and-now experiences of families and young children. I want to bridge another reality to the mix: Most practices we use to support families do not meet people's rich, diverse sociocultural needs. I want to keep this last reality in mind as I work to break free from oppressive paradigms while recognizing that you and I live within this unjust system. We need reimbursement for services and to practice within our knowledge base. With this in mind, how can we, as providers, think of comprehensive ways to support families? Can we meet the individual mental health needs of the caregiver while also meeting those of the child? Can an anti-oppressive approach help us to bridge the gap?

ABOUT THE BOOK

My proposal in this text is that training providers in the intersection of PMH, early relational health, and play therapy can aid in lowering the toll of families falling through the cracks. The book offers a framework for partnering with families to support them at one of the most vulnerable periods in life. When we identify and provide support early, we can prevent long-term adverse consequences for caregivers and children. We want to support families early and, most importantly, ensure that our intervention is culturally appropriate. The key to creating long-term changes rests on properly supporting clinicians. Proper support entails creating and stretching a capacity to think outside of colonial ways of practice that tell us to *stay in our lane*. My lane is justice and liberation. My guiding star is attuning to the needs of the person I am serving. What is yours?

The rest of this book is divided into four sections: Establishing the framework, conducting assessments, providing treatment, and transitioning out of counseling. Each section contains areas for providers to engage in critical self-reflection on their work. I encourage readers to pause and engage in the reflections and worksheets provided. Critical self-reflection can support moving beyond knowing information to embodying it. This text is a tool for supporting clinicians to collaborate with perinatal clients and their children. It is not a substitute for training and supervision from a provider with lived experience. Instead, it is a list of items I wish had been accessible when I began my work as a clinician. I hope this book builds upon how providers approach the perinatal period and the attachment relationship. May it be of benefit.

YOUR PROVIDER JOURNEY

1. What was your journey to becoming a therapist? Notice how your identities influenced your experience of becoming and being a provider.

    _____

    _____

    _____

2. How does anti-racism and anti-oppression show up in your life?

    _____

    _____

    _____

3. How connected do you feel to yourself and to your work?

_____

_____

_____

4. What is the heart and soul of your work?

_____

_____

_____

5. What would you like to shift about how you sit with families?

_____

_____

_____

6. Were you familiar with the Tenets before reading Chapter 1? If so, how have they shifted your work? If not, please take a second to review them again and notice what comes up for you. What about the Tenets are you already integrating into your work?

_____

_____

_____

REFERENCES

American Society of Anesthesiologists. (2022, October 22). Systemic racism plays role in much higher maternal mortality rate among Black women. https://tinyurl.com/pk6dddhr

Cénat, J. M. (2020). How to provide anti-racist mental health care. *Lancet*, (7)11, 929–932. https://doi.org/10.1016/S2215-0366(20)30309-6

Kendi, I. X. (2019). *How to be an antiracist*. Random House Publishing Group.

Menjivar, J. (2022, December 19). What does it mean to decolonize mental health? https://tinyurl.com/y5p32t2b

Montero, M., & Sonn, C. C. (Eds.). (2009). *Psychology of liberation: Theory and practice*. Springer.

Native Governance Center. (2021). Beyond land acknowledgment: A guide. https://nativegov.org/wp-content/uploads/2021/10/Beyond-Land-Acknowledgment_A-Guide-2021-09.pdf

Opoku-Agyeman, A. G. (Ed.). (2022). *The Black agenda*. St. Martin's Press.

Tenets Initiative. (2018). Diversity-informed tenets for work with infants, children & families/Principios informados en la diversidad para trabajar con bebés, niños, niñas y familias. Irving Harris Foundation. https://diversityinformedtenets.org/download-the-tenets/

SECTION II

Establishing the Framework

CHAPTER TWO

Grounding the Relational Approach to Therapy

Think about the work with perinatal caregivers and families as supporting an ecosystem. Family members interact with each other and navigate its environment daily. A shift in one part of the system will impact the rest. Each environment may have similar characteristics, but we recognize the vast differences and intersecting networks as we enter their system. We can understand each structure's subtle and robust differences through gentle exploration. We can learn how each piece of the system interacts with the others and the environment's unique characteristics. Non-intrusive exploration can help us avoid becoming a threat to the ecosystem's well-being. Our emotional life is similar to an ecosystem. How we navigate our world depends on the systems we interact with, the quality of those interactions, and our specific needs. Providers partner with families by entering their ecosystem. How we explore and intervene can support wellness when attuned to individual needs. A lack of attunement or interaction that does not take in the specific characteristics of that family and the individuals involved can lead to disruption and risk. I am bringing a lens of social justice, healing, and liberation into the theories that shape my practice and life experience. The heart of this framework is authenticity and collaboration. I hope anti-oppressive theory (AOT) can provide you with enough flexibility to bring your gifts, voice, and way of being into meeting the unique needs of the populations you support. This chapter provides an overview of the theoretical framework supporting work with perinatal families, babies, and young children.

DOI: 10.4324/9781003286394-4

THEORETICAL FRAMEWORK

Applying one theory through a singular lens to all families can unintentionally lead providers into an all-or-nothing way of thinking. Providers can then classify behaviors outside the expected theoretical norms as pathological and interact with families as such. This chapter invites providers to move away from the idea that difference means bad or wrong. This all-or-nothing view aligns with ethnocentrism and is central to colonization and white supremacy. Ethnocentrism is the tendency to view one's culture, values, and beliefs as most important, thereby scaling others based on our in-group (Oeberst & Matschke, 2017). This tendency does not happen consciously; it occurs outside our awareness and shows up in our interactions and how we perceive others. A decolonized, anti-racist, and anti-oppressive movement honors the diverse ways humans navigate the world. Different is sacred. Practicing clinical work from the lens that families and individuals hold lived expertise and that caregivers know their children best means we must allow space for curiosity beyond judgment. *Judgment* is the poison that pollutes the clinical relationship and, without critical change, the family's ecosystem. Curiosity supports providers in partnering with clients to understand together instead of bringing a set of prescribed answers.

Object relations theory, attachment theory, and child-centered play therapy are the three main theoretical foundations for how I work with families, a framework I call perinatal relational therapy. Anti-oppressive theory (AOT) is the filter through which we can modify and break free from Westernized and dominant ways of practice. An anti-oppressive lens helps me connect with each of the theories in my own way as I partner with families to make sense of what works for them. Since our perspective influences how we experience the world and present interventions, we can say that we put our sauce and spice into everything we do. My motto here is to take what works and leave what does not. I encourage you to do the same throughout this text.

ANTI-OPPRESSIVE THEORY (AOT)

AOT is part of a continuum of critical theoretical frameworks that seek to raise awareness of the effects of racism, exploitation, and dominance on colonized communities (Clifford, 2016). AOT asserts that imbalances in power dynamics lead to harm and calls for providers to examine power differentials in the therapist–client dynamic. The differentials include intersectional identities and the accompanying attitudes, values, and beliefs present for the provider, client, and system. *Intersectionality* is a theory that refers to how marginalized identities, like race, gender, religion, and body size, intersect with each other and face societal barriers (Crenshaw, 1991). The theory derived from the study of Black women's experiences of navigating systems like employment and law. Intersectionality is crucial for providers to recognize, as barriers and access to resources directly impact well-being. Imbalances in power dynamics frequently lead to dominant groups benefiting at the expense of others.

For example, generational wealth is connected to owning land. In the U.S.A., like many other industrialized countries, the land was stolen from Indigenous peoples by colonizers. Colonizers then went on to redistribute property and instill laws that maintained property in the hands of White communities and away from Black and Brown folk. While access to wealth does not mean freedom from suffering, it is a protective factor in life. It impacts the resources we can acquire, such as having a roof over our heads and being able to afford high-quality childcare. The legacy of colonization is present in every aspect of life. When it comes to the development of the mental health field, history reflects most research conducted by, for, and with members of dominant communities. Structural racism leads to a lack of research conducted by, for, and with minoritized communities, resulting in missing, erasing, and misconstruing integral aspects of our ecosystems. The theory of intersectionality offers a way to understand the complex layers of oppression and privilege in society and relationships. Practicing through an AOT framework moves providers to examine how they make meaning of their world, themselves, and the field (Thomas & Green, 2019).

Individuals navigating mental health systems face exposure to Eurocentric care that might be discriminatory and oppressive (Strier & Biyamin, 2014). Individualistic values like autonomy and self-determination dominate mental health theories and interventions in the U.S.A. Most evidence-based practices do not account for Indigenous healing or practices that connect with the collective, ancestors, and the earth, which are vital to many Black and Brown communities. This lack of inclusion leaves aside the needs of the global majority. As a result, clients with intersecting marginalized identities experience oppression when seeking support. When providers, especially those of us holding dominant identities, can recognize the imbalance of power present when we offer a culturally misattuned intervention, we can change how we practice and support healing. The heart of AOT is to seek what works for the client with attention to the past and present. A tool for applying AOT is the lens of cultural humility.

Cultural humility is an anti-oppressive practice that arose from observations that learning about another person's culture through attending cultural competency courses or workshops was harmful (Tervalon & Murray-Garcia, 1998). This practice calls for providers to reflect critically and critique their values, beliefs, and experiences. Through critical reflection, providers examine their worldview for biases, dominant perspectives, and other harmful material. Biases can be explicit and implicit (Bruster et al., 2019). Explicit refers to stances providers knowingly endorse or declare. Believing that Black and Brown immigrants and refugees are in the U.S.A. to take *our* jobs is an example of an explicit bias. Implicit biases are unconscious harmful beliefs about people outside one's cultural group. For instance, white supremacy is a racist ideology where people with lighter skin believe they hold superiority over other races and skin tones (Anti-Defamation League, n.d.). This belief system infiltrates everything we come into contact with, including policies, practices, and how humans might interact with each other. White supremacy, colonization, and structural racism are interrelated. Their deep impact on how people navigate the world often leads communities to align with whiteness.

Alignment with whiteness shows up in Latin America and many other Black and Brown communities as colorism, a form of oppression where those with lighter skin are privileged over darker skin tones. Due to the complexity of white supremacy and the nature of implicit biases, members of historically marginalized communities can hold prejudices against our in-groups, as in the case of colorism, anti-blackness, and anti-indigeneity (Staats et al., 2015). A Latin American immigrant may hold implicit biases against other Latin American immigrants due to their phenotype or country of origin. These beliefs are often stereotypical and develop over time "due to certain cultural groups being paired with specific characteristics" (Bruster et al., 2019, p. 655). Here is another example. An implicit bias from a provider from religious group A might unintentionally lead that provider to judge a family from religious group B. The provider might erroneously view certain behaviors, dynamics, and strengths integral to the family's religion as harmful. If judgments go unexamined, the therapist might harm the family through microaggressions and misattuned treatment recommendations. Microaggressions are subtle, verbal, and non-verbal put-downs about people belonging to racial, ethnic, and other historically marginalized groups (Hook et al., 2016).

The second step in practicing cultural humility is engaging in self-critique. Critique is a process of examination that helps providers increase privilege awareness (Rosen et al., 2017). Privilege refers to holding dominant identities that do not face social exclusion, like heterosexual and cisgender identities. Using the example above, the provider might find it helpful to examine how dominant views on religion impact families from non-dominant religious groups. Critique is vital for understanding the limits of knowledge and perception. Through critique, providers can take an other-oriented frame focusing on collaborating and understanding the family's experience. This step moves providers away from ethnocentrism to centering the other's experience. Cultural humility shifts providers out of the expert role and into a space of curiosity. As providers step outside their expertise, they can learn to rely on the client's lived experience as the true expert.

The starting point for building client collaboration is a critical look at the therapist's value system. A critical assessment can help providers understand how societal discourses and systemic racism contribute to our conceptualization of pathology. Figure 2.1 shows how structural racism informs institutions like

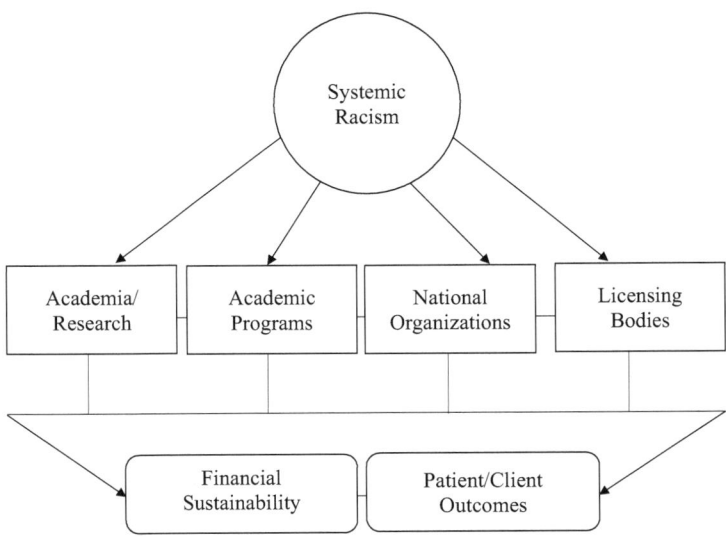

FIGURE 2.1 Systemic Racism, Training, and Goals

academia, academic programs, national organizations, and licensing bodies and goals like financial sustainability and patient outcomes. The point here is to illustrate how biases filter into every area of practice, and no one is immune from them.

No one practice will culturally attune to everyone. Through the engagement of curiosity and humility on the provider's part, therapeutic collaboration can become a space for healing and belonging. It is essential to say that although I am calling providers to engage in anti-oppressive practices, this does not mean that clients will automatically lean into collaboration. The trust the individual shares or chooses not to share with us will depend on multiple complex factors for which they owe us no explanation. Those reasons might include historical trauma in the medical field and past relationships with providers or interactions with individuals without lived experience in different intersectional identities. In this sense, cultural humility supports providers in recognizing limits and responsibility. Our responsibility as providers is to do the work; the limit is that what we do will never be enough. Engagement in anti-oppressive and anti-racist work will never make us fully competent or equip us with all the skills to navigate and repair all relationships. Nevertheless, we have a sacred duty to reflect, critique, and actively rebel against all sources of oppression.

I am presenting three clinical theories that are the basis of my training and experience with clients: Object relations theory (ORT), attachment theory (AT), and child-directed play therapy (CDPT). A comprehensive discussion of each theory's intricacies is beyond this text's scope. Readers will find ORT, AT, and CDPT filtered through the lens of AOT.

OBJECT RELATIONS THEORY: A PSYCHODYNAMIC APPROACH

Psychodynamic or psychoanalytic therapies assert that the root of emotional distress is unconscious motivations (Safran, 2012). Therapists in this school of psychotherapeutic thought support clients' awareness of the unconscious material contributing to emotional distress and disturbance to functioning. The vehicle for support is talk therapy, where the provider listens and makes connections between the client's communications (verbal and non-verbal) and experiences. Although there is no unified theory for the psychodynamic approach, the therapist's interpretations aim to help the individual embrace complexity and tolerate ambiguity. Life is rarely one-sided. Many distinctive intersecting aspects shape who we are and how we think and feel. By understanding some of our layered roots of distress, healing can begin to happen. Object relations theory (ORT) is a psychodynamic framework exploring the rich and complex world of relationships that we carry within ourselves (Applegate, 1990). As mentioned earlier, most psychological interventions were created without the input of Black and Brown communities. Many psychoanalytical approaches have been dangerous and discriminatory to minoritized communities such as BIPOC and LGBTQ+ folk (Belkin & White, 2020). AOT reminds us that the past influences the present, and naming history is vital to healing. As such, I will layer anti-racist and anti-oppressive practices into my conceptualization of ORT, as failure to do so can lead to harm and further oppression.

A foundational premise of ORT is that people develop internalized mental representations of themselves and others (Frankland, 2010). Mental representations are ideas, beliefs, or fantasies outside of conscious awareness. We use the term *outside of conscious awareness* because, similar to implicit biases, the person is usually unaware of the internalized representations and their impact on feelings and interactions. ORT can help us understand the caregivers' experience, concerns, and transition to *caregiverhood*. Klein, Fairbairn, and Winnicott are among the many analysts who have influenced the framework of ORT. Each analyst brought a lens through which providers might understand psychopathology and the client's presentation. I take a middle-ground approach to ORT, borrowing from different perspectives but with a sharp focus on AOT and believing that a human's primary motivation is a connection to others.

ORT suggests that people have two levels of relationships: One with the internal world and the other with the external (Frankland, 2010). Internal objects are the unconscious representations of self and others, while external objects refer to the actual people in our environment and life. Internal objects impact relationships with external objects, which means that what we believe about ourselves and the world influences and may distort our perception and worldview. For example, during pregnancy, a birthing person might begin creating ideas of what they imagine their child will be like. The pregnant person might think the baby will have specific characteristics like easygoing, energetic, creative, and so on. When the baby joins the family, the caregiver might have other internal representations of the child. These representations are what we call object representation or fantasy. The caregiver's object representation will influence how the caregiver experiences and relates to the child. That is to say that the caregiver's perception of their child is unconsciously filtered through the lens of their inner world. In this way, the caregiver might unintentionally develop a relationship with their imagined perception of the child rather than the child. Consider times in counseling when an individual might make statements about former loved ones (i.e., long-term romantic relationships, parent–child relationships, etc.) such as, *"They never saw me for me," "They wanted me to be someone else,"* or *"They were not interested in me, what I like, or who I was."*

Object representations are an active influence on how we think and behave. Warped views of reality can lead to intense emotional distress (Frankland, 2010). Without support, emotional distress can affect interpersonal relationships. A young child abused by their primary caregiver might begin to internalize a sense that they are bad. Badness might become their self-representation. *"I am not good enough," "no one cares about me,"* and *"I am bad"* may be a part of identity and how that child views themselves. The child might also internalize a representation of their caregiver, perhaps as destructive, dangerous, or scary. As the child grows up, they might perceive danger and destruction from others and behave accordingly. The expression of behavior will depend on neurobiological and environmental factors and might differ from person to person. On a spectrum, individuals might either internalize or externalize feelings into behaviors. In our example, danger and destruction are now one aspect of that individual's object representation or fantasy. The fantasy of others as dangerous is present in the person's mind regardless of whether situations are safe. During parenthood, the person's self-representation of being bad may translate into believing they are a bad parent and that the baby also knows this and rejects the caregiver because of it. The caregiver may experience distress when they perceive their child dislikes them and their self-representation as "bad." Without proper support, distress may increase, influencing the caregiver's and child's mental health outcomes, including their relational well-being.

We recognize that the world is not a safe place for most individuals, especially those of us with historically marginalized identities. An internal sense of safety or being able to build a network of safe relationships becomes more complicated when we experience early childhood adversity in the context of caregiver relationships (Zeanah, 2019). It is vital to note that the compounding of systemic barriers contributes to feelings of badness. Humans hold relationships with their environment, including nature, the elements, and climate. When families cannot access the resources needed to meet basic needs, overall well-being declines. Providers working from an anti-oppressive lens must identify how societal barriers impact the family's well-being and the perinatal caregiver's inner world. Considering that pathology resides inside the individual and within relationships without understanding how mezzo, macro, and metta systems impact families can lead to providers erroneously conceptualizing oppression as living in the person's mental world instead of being a societal barrier. The lack of consideration for the impact of colonization and structural racism is one of the major criticisms of psychodynamic theories (Belkin & White, 2020). Providers with dominant identities must take special care in understanding historical trauma and present-day barriers that impact minoritized communities. Many communities do not experience time as linear but rather in cycles. A cyclical view of time acknowledges that the "past" and "future" are with us at each moment (Chisholm Hatfield et al., 2018). When painful events are part of our ancestor's journey, they are present with us and in how we experience the world. Structural racism, poverty, unpaid family leave, and inaccessible childcare costs are just a few barriers harming caregivers and babies, especially members of historically marginalized communities.

Clinical Applications

In ORT, the caregiver's understanding of their child's behavior ties back to the family of origin and the caregiver's earliest relationships. Applying cultural humility helps providers to acknowledge the limits of clinical training and to account for clients' lived expertise.

ORT holds that a baby's self-understanding begins in relationships (Clarke et al., 2008). The baby thoroughly relies on their caregivers and does not experience themself as a person or as being separate from others. This concept of the baby as connected to others is the heart of Winnicott's famous quote, "There is no such thing as a baby" (Winnicott, 1975, p. 99). Winnicott explained that when one sees a baby there is always a caregiver. Bring to mind the image of a baby chestfeeding. As the baby eats, they might make eye contact and reach for the caregiver. These moments of reaching might be the beginning of the baby's perception of the caregiver as separate from the baby, forming the start of a self-representation. The baby begins the process of knowing that the caregiver can meet their needs. As they reach with their hands and touch their caregiver, we can think of the baby saying, "*You are still here with me.*" We also have a person beginning to relate to their child and developing their identity as a caregiver. Building an identity as a caregiver can shift with each child joining the family. The caregiver might give meaning to the behavior as the baby feeds, looks away, or reaches. The caregiver's object relations will influence their perception of the baby. The meaning of the behavior will depend on the intersection of object relations and environmental stressors. We can conceptualize object relations on a scale from self-destructive to self-affirming. For instance, the caregiver might interpret the baby reaching with their hands during feeding as *"My baby loves me," "The baby knows that I have no idea what I'm doing,"* or *"They are hitting me already."* Therapists partner with clients to understand their history, inner world, and narratives.

Distressing experiences can create false, disturbed views of self. The *false self* is the wall we develop to protect ourselves from others (Winnicott, 1975). Distorted object relations can lead the individual to have an all-or-nothing view of self and others, leading to distress. We then navigate the world filtering experience through our false self-representation. The walls defend us from an innate fear of destruction arising from our lived experience. A caregiver who was physically abused as a child might develop a fantasy that they can only relate to others through aggression and control (Seligman, 1999). I invite us to consider ancestral lineage as we conceptualize "lived experience."

We carry our history and those who came before us within us. The false self can give us a distorted sense of control over life. A caregiver with complex developmental trauma might view their baby's behavior, such as crying, as a signal that they are a terrible parent. In a way, believing that the crying is "their fault" gives a sense of power over the situation. The caregiver might think, *"If I do things just right, this will stop."* The sense of power is a fantasy, as babies can cry even after caregivers meet their physical and emotional needs. The problem happens when the caregiver believes that the behavior should stop or be different with their intervention and that, when it is not, the fantasy of being bad arises or strengthens. By filtering this theory through an AOT lens, we can think of the false self as protective, something within ourselves worth honoring instead of something to eradicate from our being. We can think of the false self as adaptive for members of communities fighting for survival. Shifting the relationship with ourselves requires understanding historical and present-day systems of oppression. Using the example above, I invite you to think about the intersection of the child welfare system with the lives of Black, Brown, and Indigenous peoples. For a caregiver of Color, self-representation intertwines with a history of transgenerational trauma, including the trafficking of humans during chattel slavery and the stealing of Indigenous children from families and placement into residential schools.

In the early relational health field, we use the term "keeping the baby in mind." This concept "refers to the capacity of the parents [caregivers] to experience the baby as an 'intentional' being rather than simply viewing him or her [them] in terms of physical characteristics or behaviour" (Barlow & Svanberg,

2009, p. 6). As caregivers experience the baby as an intentional being, they begin giving meaning to the baby's behaviors. Meaning-making influences the choices the caregiver makes as they consider the impact of those choices on the baby's experience. However, the caregiver's interpretation of the baby is connected to the caregiver's object relations. I view the role of adulthood as a time for humans to become loving, responsive, and compassionate caregivers to ourselves. In counseling, the therapist partners with the client in understanding internalized relationships. Through the experience of being seen and heard in collaboration with the therapist, the client can begin to internalize a different way of relating to their caregiving role (Frankland, 2010).

ATTACHMENT THEORY: TAKING A CULTURAL LENS

Many therapy modalities use attachment theory to understand psychopathology in the caregiver, child, and their relationship. When working with perinatal caregivers and their little ones, attachment theory (AT) can be a lens that helps providers maintain the child's needs present in counseling.

I present AT through a lens that recognizes the individuality among the families and cultures in our communities. By individuality, I mean the differences in relating, interacting, teaching, and disciplining of children present among diverse groups. One of the most important lessons I have learned through an anti-oppressive framework is that applying one technique or theory to everyone can lead to harm. Harm can take place because individuals, families, and our world are not one-dimensional. Attunement and sensitivity can present differently among individuals from different cultures. Humans are complex in ways that can be incomprehensible to others outside our cultural circles. Providers must understand the meaning of observable behaviors through a collaborative relationship with the family.

A Brief History of Attachment Theory

Founded by Bowlby, AT posits that individuals are born with an intrinsic biological motivation towards relationships (Bowlby, 1982). The theory proposes that a baby's innate drive is to make meaningful relationships with caregivers as an adaptation to survival. The baby's instinctual responses activate protective reactions in their primary caregivers. Primary caregivers become attachment figures for the child. AT stems from the psychoanalytic school of object relations and holds some overlap (Priel & Besser, 2001). Bowlby shifted away from psychoanalytic thought and ORT and into the world of instinct theories. Some analysts conceptualize AT as an object relation where the baby begins to internalize a sense of the caregiver. However, as proposed by Bowlby, AT focuses on the impact of real-life relationships and events the child experiences through an ethological lens rather than relationships with internalized representations (Ainsworth & Bowlby, 1991). Ethology refers to the study of animal behavior.

AT proposes that behaviors like crying, smiling, and following are adaptive responses to the activation of the child's attachment system (Ainsworth & Bowlby, 1991). The attachment system is a biologically based group of behaviors that activates when the baby is under stress. Discomfort moves the child to seek closeness from their attachment figure. The responsive behaviors demonstrated by the primary caregiver when the baby is distressed can help the child build an internalized sense of safety and trust. Caregiver sensitivity provides a secure base to which the child can return in moments of distress. The repeated experiences with the caregiver help the child develop an internal working model (IWM), a mental representation of relationships. IWM and object representations are parallel constructs (Priel & Besser, 2001). ORT holds that internal representations or fantasies are present in every interaction. Fantasy impacts how we perceive a situation. In counseling, we want to understand how the caregiver's object relations affect their view of the child and of themselves as a caregiver. IWM, on the other hand, helps individuals set expectations about their world and others, thereby guiding attachment-related behaviors. The caregiver's attunement to their child steers what the baby learns to expect from the world.

Attachment is present in the context of multiple close relationships. However, the mother–child relationship has been the focus of most research. Mary Ainsworth helped expand AT through her study of families in Uganda and Baltimore. Her findings led to the development of the Strange Situation Procedure, a method for assessing and categorizing the attachment relationship between mothers and babies. Ainsworth classified attachment as either secure, resistant, or avoidant. In 1990, Main and Solomon identified disorganized attachment as a fourth category. Ainsworth pinpointed the importance of a sensitive and responsive caregiver as vital to developing a secure attachment.

Critical Lens

Critics argue that AT has yet to go through the level of expansion and development that some scholars have given to other psychological theories (Dawson, 2018; Keller, 2021; Stern et al., 2022). We know that the need for expansion and liberation is true for most if not all psychological theories. The past is a key to understanding the present. This section presents a brief synopsis of the development of AT so that readers can critically reflect on its environmental and historical lens. Engaging in this practice can place the theory in our current context and that of the families we support. An intentional look at the history of AT highlights the erasure of historically marginalized communities.

Bowlby's conceptualization of AT began forming as the world recovered from WWII. One of Bowlby's most pivotal papers was published in 1952 by the World Health Organization (WHO) and addressed the effects of abandoned and orphaned children (Bowlby, 1952). In the U.S.A., the 1950s and 1960s reflected a time of great concern regarding gender roles, including traditional roles of mothers and women in the workforce (Keller, 2021). Foundational observations and studies in AT engaged Caucasian middle-class mothers and their babies as participants, leaving out individuals of Color, people living in poverty, and many other communities. From 1954 to 1955, Mary Ainsworth collected data from observations and interpreter-facilitated interviews of 26 mothers across 23 households in Uganda (Ainsworth, 1967). The analysis of that data paved the way for developing the Strange Situation Procedure, a tool for establishing, researching, and organizing attachment patterns. The observations Ainsworth made in Uganda and her subsequent studies of mother–baby dyads in the U.S.A. helped frame AT as cross-cultural and universally applicable.

Acquiring a copy of Ainsworth's book *Infancy in Uganda: Infant care and the growth of love* was challenging, as it is out of print. This book holds Ainsworth's original narrations and analysis of the Ugandan observations and is often cited in the AT literature to this day. Before we continue, I invite us to reflect deeply on the dynamics of a White woman from outside Ugandan culture sitting in people's households with a translator and a notepad. I wonder what it was like for the families to be observed. What was their felt experience? I am curious about giving behavior meaning without profoundly understanding the sociocultural context. To understand behavior from an anti-oppressive framework, we must know its context and what it means to the caregiver. Without that context and collaboration, we risk applying ethnocentric interpretations and harming the populations we seek to support.

As a clinician, I can lean on AT to consider the importance of relationships to the baby's development but must consider the caregiver's expertise as a guide to the work. This shift of the caregiver as an expert is a challenge in society and fields that center the professional's expertise. A central premise of AT is that sensitive and responsive caregiving is vital to developing a secure attachment. We have lists of caregiver behaviors that lead to certain attachment types and other lists of child behaviors that signal which attachment type is present. The danger here falls on researchers' and providers' definitions of sensitivity and responsiveness. The current understanding of attachment behaviors and types holds a Eurocentric lens.

Let us wonder together:

- Is face-to-face contact between a caregiver and their baby vital in every culture? What about the caregiver's vocalizations to the baby, like talking, singing, and reading?

- What about a child raised in a culture where caregivers do not frequently verbalize the words "I love you?" Do they experience harm?
- If a community or family is not demonstrating behaviors perceived as attachment-building in the West, does that mean their culture lacks childrearing skills and hurts the child's development?
- Is the caregiver then insensitive and the child at risk for insecure attachment?

Exploration and proximity-seeking are two other cornerstones of AT. As the baby explores their environment, they move away from their caregiver and return when stress increases. In the U.S.A., cultural values of independence, self-actualization, and autonomy influence what providers consider appropriate levels of exploration. Continuing our reflective process:

- Do cultures encouraging the child's dependence on the caregiver harm the child or their capacity to build relationships?
- What about cultures that keep the child close by, baby-wearing most of the day or snuggling the baby in a moss bag or cradleboard?

Theoretical ethnocentrism is dangerous. It can lead providers and systems to create oppressive interventions and policies. What I hope you get out of this section is a sense that there is no "right way" for a caregiver to raise and love their child. It should go without saying, but I am not talking about abusive practices like beating or ignoring a child altogether. In 2021, I attended a training called Positive Indian Parenting through the National Indian Child Welfare Association. The trainers encouraged participants to consider how families related to and disciplined their children before colonization. Attention to the impact of transgenerational traumas like colonization, chattel slavery, and genocide is vital in maintaining an AOT framework. I am focusing on how individuals show up worldwide and inviting providers to partner with families to understand behaviors and relationships. The conceptualization of AT presented here is one where relationships are vital to the child's well-being, but how those relationships show up depends on each child, caregiver, and family. Through this lens, providers are, again, invited to embrace complexity and tolerate ambiguity. Cultural humility entails sitting with the not knowing.

CHILD-DIRECTED PLAY THERAPY

Child-directed play therapy (CDPT) focuses on centering the client's needs by providing a nondirective, nonjudgmental, and accepting space (Guerney, 2001; Ray & Landreth, 2019; Velasquez, 2022). The nature of CDPT involves toys and a space that allows the client to choose the direction of the therapy, including activities and interactions with the provider. Foundational literary works in CDPT emphasized the need for the therapist to follow the lead of the child's manipulation of toys and narrative, suggesting the strategy to be applicable for children able to do imaginative play, generally aged 3 and above. Dr. Courtney (2020) coined the term *infant play therapy*, referring to play therapy models for babies and young children. Infant play therapy can include current play therapy models adjusted for infant populations, early relational health models that engage play, and new play therapy models specific to infants and young children. When I think of infant-directed play therapy, I imagine a framework where the caregiver is attuned to their child's needs and playfully engages them. For interactions to be baby-led, the caregiver must center what their child might need and feel in the moment. The provider is a gentle observer and collaborator who accepts what the dyad reflects and provides the experience of being seen and heard.

Clinical Applications of CDPT

Guerney (2001) outlined five principles that differentiate nondirective play therapy from other forms. I will use Guerney's tenets to support the conceptualization of this model for babies and young children.

Principle 1: The child directs the therapy. Therapists observe the child's interactions and movements and the caregiver's responses and needs. CDPT supports interactions that meet the client's needs while considering the child's developmental stage. This nondirective way of being holds an AOT lens, as the provider avoids introducing ideas, games, and other activities.

Principle 2: The provider focuses on the child's inner world instead of presenting problems. Babies and young children are developing an internalized sense of self (IWM) that happens in the context of caregiving relationships. To center the child's world, providers support caregivers in mentalizing their child. A caregiver's mentalization refers to their capacity to reflect on and imagine how the baby thinks and feels about the relationship and situations (Luyten et al., 2017). How a caregiver thinks about their child will depend on multiple cultural contexts.

Principle 3: The provider accepts the child's reality. Providers work with caregivers to *see the child the caregiver sees*. In this precept, therapists engage in a parallel process where they mentalize the caregiver, and the caregiver mentalizes their child. Providers must be aware of their judgments and concerns regarding the right way to be and play with a child.

Principle 4: CDPT is not a set of guidelines that providers follow. Instead, it is a system of observing and honoring the other's reality.

Principle 5: The provider avoids centering techniques like psychoeducation or structured activities into the caregiver–child interactions. We might bring ideas to support caregiver–baby interactions and encourage the dyad to find their individual flow.

A RELATIONAL APPROACH IN ACTION

My approach to working with perinatal families is relational and anti-oppressive. This framework targets the emotional changes during the transition to caregiverhood with a lens on how systemic barriers impact well-being. Becoming a caregiver can trigger or exacerbate underlying mental health complications. Through the therapy, providers can partner with families to understand internal narratives that the caregiver might be carrying. Understanding internal narratives is vital to the family's overall well-being, as it can impact how the caregivers interact with themselves and with their children. This relational approach honors that the most significant contributor to complications is the effects of racism, colonization, and other forms of oppression. As such, providers utilize cultural humility to consistently examine feelings that arise as they interact with families. Chapter 5 discusses reflective practice at length. A dual process in therapy involves supporting the caregiver while keeping the child's needs present. As providers interact with families, they observe the dynamics between them and their children. Interpretations of observations come from the caregiver, the expert on their child. The provider encourages positive interactions that are mutually satisfying to the baby and the caregiver by understanding what behaviors mean to the caregiver. Perinatal relational therapy holds five guidelines for working with families:

1. Structural racism, colonization, and oppression are the most significant contributors to perinatal mental health complications.
2. Object relations impact the transition to parenthood and may worsen mental health symptoms.
3. Integrating babies and young children when treating perinatal caregivers is vital to their well-being.
4. Interactions between caregivers and children have deep cultural meanings, which we can understand through the family's interpretation.
5. An AOT view of relationships includes those we hold with the environment, elements, climate, ancestors, and descendants, among others.

CONCLUSION

Supporting families during the perinatal period requires attunement to their specific needs. How a provider attunes must culturally match the caregiver's and baby's needs. The provider's capacity to connect with the caregiver and provide supportive care will depend on their capacity to hold an anti-racist and anti-oppressive lens in their conceptualization of psychopathology. Perinatal relational therapy posits that a caregiver's internal world can impact their relationships with others. ORT offers a tool for understanding the caregiver's inner narratives and how they may or may not correlate with the external world. A cultural lens to AT supports providers in seeing how the caregiver relates to their child and meets their needs. AT serves as a guide to meeting the specific needs of infants and young children while supporting caregivers. Nondirective play supports interactions without making changes or recommendations that might be stressful for the family.

Your Theoretical Framework

The training you have acquired throughout your career is valuable to supporting communities. When integrating new theoretical frameworks, it is helpful to briefly assess what is already in your toolbox. Think about it as building knowledge on top of knowledge.

The questions below can help you examine your clinical skills and how to apply an anti-oppressive and relational lens to your knowledge base.

1. What theories inform your practice?

    _____

    _____

    _____

2. Please apply a critical lens to answering the following questions: What is the history behind each theory? Consider the social location of founders and researchers and the sociopolitical context during the theory's development.

    _____

    _____

    _____

3. What adaptations have you and/or other providers made to integrate an anti-oppressive lens into the theories?

    _____

    _____

    _____

4. How does each theory apply to working with perinatal people? Babies and young children? And the caregiver–child relationship?
    *   If you identified gaps, what dominant and non-dominant sources can support your learning?

    _____

    _____

    _____

5. How do the theories and their interventions align with the Tenets?

    _____

    _____

    _____

6. How are you expanding the view of relationships beyond the lens of person-to-person interactions (i.e., nature, spiritual, animals, the elements, climate)?

    _____

    _____

    _____

REFERENCES

Ainsworth, M. D. S. (1967). *Infancy in Uganda: Infant care and the growth of love.* Johns Hopkins Press.

Ainsworth, M. D. S., & Bowlby, J. (1991). An ethological approach to personality development. *American Psychologist, 46*(4), 333–341. https://doi.org/10.1037/0003-066X.46.4.333

Anti-Defamation League. (n.d.) White supremacy. https://extremismterms.adl.org/glossary/white-supremacy

Applegate, J. S. (1990). Theory, culture, and behavior: Object relations in context. *Child & Adolescent Social Work Journal, 7*(2), 85–100. https://doi.org/10.1007/bf00757647

Barlow, J., & Svanberg, P. O. (2009). *Keeping the baby in mind: Infant mental health in practice.* Taylor & Francis.

Belkin, M., & White, M. (Eds.). (2020). *Intersectionality and relational psychoanalysis.* Routledge.

Bowlby, J. (1952). Maternal care and mental health: A report on behalf of the World Health Organization as a contribution to the United Nations programme for the welfare of homeless children. World Health Organization.

Bowlby, J. (1982). *Attachment and loss: Attachment* (2nd edition, Vol 1). Basic Books.

Bruster, B. E., Lane, T. Y., & Smith, B. D. (2019). Challenging implicit bias: Preparing students to practice with African American families. *Social Work Education, 38*(5), 654–665. https://doi.org/10.1080/02615479.2019.1594753

Chisholm Hatfield, S., Marino, E., Whyte, K. P., Dello, K. D., & Mote, P. W. (2018). Indian time: Time, seasonality, and culture in Traditional Ecological Knowledge of climate change. *Ecological Process, 7*(25). https://doi.org/10.1186/s13717-018-0136-6

Clarke, S., Hahn, H., & Hoggett, P. (Eds.). (2008). *Object relations and social relations: The implications of relational turn in psychoanalysis.* Karnac.

Clifford, D. (2016). Oppression and professional ethics. *Ethics and Social Welfare*, *10*(1), 4–18. https://doi.org/10.1080/17496535.2015.1072225

Courtney, J. A. (Ed.). (2020). *Infant play therapy*. Routledge.

Crenshaw, K. W. (1991). Mapping the margins: Intersectionality, identity politics, and violence against women of color. https://www.racialequitytools.org/resource files/mapping-margins.pdf

Dawson, N. K. (2018). From Uganda to Baltimore to Alexandra Township: How far can Ainsworth's theory stretch? *South African Journal of Psychiatry*, *24*, 1–8. https://doi.org/10.4102/sajpsychiatry.v24i0.1137

Frankland, A. G. (2010). *The little psychotherapy book: Object relations in practice*. Oxford University Press.

Guerney, L. (2001). Child-centered play therapy. *International Journal of Play Therapy*, *10*(2), 13–31. https://doi.org/10.1037/h0089477

Hook, J. N., Farrell, J. E., Davis, D. E., DeBlaere, C., Van Tongeren, D. R., & Utsey, S. O. (2016). Cultural humility and racial microaggressions in counseling. *Journal of Counseling Psychology*, *63*(3), 269–277. https://doi.org/10.1037/cou0000114

Keller, H. (2021). *The myth of attachment theory*. Taylor and Francis.

Luyten, P., Nijssens, L., Fonagy, P., & Mayes, L. C. (2017). Parental reflective functioning: Theory, research, and clinical applications. *The Psychoanalytic Study of the Child*, *70*(1), 174–199. https://doi.org/10.1080/00797308.2016.1277901

Main, M., & Solomon, J. (1990). Procedures for identifying infants as disorganized/ disoriented during the Ainsworth Strange Situation. In M. T. Greenberg, D. Cicchetti, & E. M. Cummings (Eds.), *Attachment in the preschool years: Theory, research, and intervention* (pp. 121–160). University of Chicago.

Oeberst, A., & Matschke, C. (2017). Word order and world order: Titles of intergroup conflicts may increase ethnocentrism by mentioning the in-group first. *Journal of Experimental Psychology: General*, *146*(5), 672–690. https://doi.org/10.1037/xge0000300.supp

Priel, B., & Besser, A. (2001). Bridging the gap between attachment and object relations theories: A study of the transition to motherhood. *British Journal of Medical Psychology*, *74*(1), 85–100. https://doi.org/10.1348/000711201160821

Ray, D., & Landreth, G. (2019). Child-centered play therapy. *Play Therapy*, *14*(3), 18–19.

Rosen, D., McCall, J., & Goodkind, S. (2017). Teaching critical self-reflection through the lens of cultural humility: An assignment in a social work diversity course. *Social Work Education*, *36*(3), 289–298. https://doi.org/10.1080/02615479.2017.1287260

Safran, J. D. (2012). *Psychoanalysis and psychoanalytic therapies*. American Psychological Association.

Seligman, S. (1999). Integrating kleinian theory and intersubjective infant research observing projective identification. *Psychoanalytic Dialogues*, *9*(2), 129–159. https://doi.org/10.1080/10481889909539311

Staats, C., Capatosto, K., Wright, R. A., & Contractor, D. (2015). State of the science: Implicit bias review 2015. Kirwan Institute. http://kirwaninstitute.osu.edu/ wp-content/uploads/2015/05/2015-Kirwan-implicit-bias.pdf

Stern, J. A., Barbarin, O., & Jude, C. (2022). Working toward anti-racist perspectives in attachment theory, research, and practice. *Attachment & Human Development*, *24*(3), 392–422. https://doi.org/10.1080/14616734.2021.1976933

Strier, R., & Biyamin, S. (2014). Introducing anti-oppressive social work practices in public services: Rhetoric to practice. *British Journal of Social Work*, *44*(8), 2095–2112. https://doi.org/10.1093/bjsw/bct049

Tervalon, M., & Murray-Garcia, J. (1998). Cultural humility versus cultural competence: A critical distinction in defining physician training outcomes in multicultural education. *Journal of Health Care for the Poor and Underserved*, *9*(2), 117–125. https://doi.org/10.1353/hpu.2010.0233

Thomas, R., & Green, J. (2019). A way of life: Indigenous perspectives on anti oppressive living. *First Peoples Child & Family Review*, *14*(1). 82–92. https://doi.org/10.7202/1069529ar

Velasquez, M. (2022). Let's go outside: Nature-based play therapy through the lens of cultural humility. In J. A. Courtney, J. Langley, L. Wonders, R. LaPiere, & R. Heiko (Eds.), *Nature-based play and expressive interventions for working with children, teens and families*. Routledge.

Winnicott, D. W. (1975). *Through paediatrics to psycho-analysis*. Basic Books.

Zeanah, C. H. (Ed.). (2019). *The handbook of infant mental health* (4th edition). The Guilford Press.

CHAPTER THREE

An Overview of the Perinatal Period

Before colonization, when a baby was born, communities would gather to celebrate life and support the new families (Farrell, 2022; First Nations Health Authority & Office of the Provincial Health Officer, 2021; Smithsonian, n.d.). Pregnancy, birth, and the postpartum period were considered unique and powerful times filled with abundance and possibilities. The birthing person received respite and care from elders and other community members as they healed from delivery and transitioned into parenthood. The family was celebrated, and support was abundant. Although these practices remain present in some communities, colonization, chattel slavery, capitalism, racism, forced migration, and poverty continuously disrupt the importance of the transition to parenthood. Colonization erased traditional practices from Indigenous communities, introducing the medicalization of birth and other Westernized practices. Capitalism impacts families through barriers like unpaid medical leave, lack of affordable care or centralized insurance, and the 40-hour work week. Racism, the legacy of chattel slavery, continues to place the lives of Black and Brown individuals at risk as they navigate the medical system. The high rates of infant and birthing person mortality reflect structural racism's impact. This chapter provides an overview of perinatal mental health (PMH) complications, systemic risk factors, and considerations for providers to practice from an AOP lens.

A LOOK AT THE PERINATAL PERIOD

Nay is back home after delivering baby Yassir four days ago. During the next two years, Yassir will develop a sense of self and connection to the world. Development takes place within the sacred space between caregiver and baby.

DOI: 10.4324/9781003286394-5

As Nay creates a sense of safety for Yassir, Nay, too, requires connection and protection. When baby Yassir was born, so was caregiver Nay. Caregiver and baby are navigating the world in different but parallel roles. Nay must protect Yassir while also making sense of this new identity as a caregiver and the changes it brings. Western society often misses supporting the birthing person as they transition into caregiverhood. Caregivers are learning how to find balance as their world suddenly changes. An internal sense of balance will look different for all parties involved, but the challenges faced increase at the intersection of marginalized identities. I learned from clients that this need to find balance exists whether the first or the sixth child joins the family, as each pregnancy and birth requires adjustment. The societal expectation is that caregivers will naturally bond with their babies, love the joy of the newborn period, and find great pleasure in their new role. In reality, babyhood and early childhood are difficult periods where people often struggle in silence.

Perinatal mood and anxiety disorders like postpartum depression are the most common childbirth complications, affecting up to one in two individuals depending on barriers and risk factors (Matthews et al., 2021). For people who experience mood and anxiety disorders, shame, guilt, and fear often rise to silence attempts at support. There is shame in the narrative, *"This is the best time of your life,"* because someone does not feel that way; they can think something is inherently wrong with them. Internalized shame rises in the presence of mental health complications. There is guilt at not feeling like a good enough caregiver, not enjoying every minute, or being resentful. There is shame in thinking that pregnancy and caregiverhood are sacred duties, only to find that we might feel numb, lost, and like we are failing at every corner. People can experience a sense of hopelessness when they think that loved ones would be more supportive, involved, or connected, only to find themselves in isolation and under increased stress. Even when people can push through these feelings and attempt to seek support, they can face significant barriers.

MEDICAL MISTRUST IN THE PERINATAL PERIOD

Medical mistrust is adaptive in BIPOC communities. It is not an unfounded fear from nowhere but a truth based on historical and present-day trauma. I often hear providers mention stigma as a reason why communities of Color have lower levels of service utilization. The narrative of stigma blurs the realities of medical abuse. For individuals with marginalized identities, stigma is connected with historical trauma. A critical question for providers to explore is: What power dynamics contributed to this outcome? Being aware of the foundation of medical distrust can support providers in connecting with clients in an attuned way.

There are many sources of information providers can reach to learn more about historical and present-day trauma, which are somewhat out of the scope of this text, but I will highlight some realities here:

- Enslaved birthing people were tortured by individuals conducting heinous experiments like cesarean sections without anesthesia.
- BIPOC communities and individuals with disabilities faced forced sterilization at different historical points.
- BIPOC individuals were subjected to forced contraceptive consumption and testing.
- For 40 years, a group of 400 Black men in Tuskegee received no treatment for syphilis so that researchers could study the condition's progression.
- In 1946 to 1948, the National Institutes of Health conducted horrendous and unethical experimentation in Guatemala. One of the lead investigators from the Tuskegee "study" led the "experimentation." Investigators infected thousands of vulnerable populations, like children in orphanages, soldiers, prisoners, and patients in mental institutions, with sexually transmitted diseases to observe the course of the illness.
- Indigenous children were kidnapped from their parents and placed into boarding schools to assimilate them into European culture and erase their Indigeneity. We are still recovering the bodies of children killed in these boarding schools.
- Propagation of the racist beliefs that Black individuals have a higher pain tolerance. This racist idea is still present in some healthcare-related books.

(Carney, 2021; National Partnership for Women & Children, 2020; Rodriguez & Garcia, 2013)

Structural racism contributes to Black birthing people dying at rates three to four times higher than their White counterparts (Owens & Fett, 2019). Although Black perinatal people experience some of the highest rates of PMH conditions, they are less likely than non-Black folk to receive care (Matthews et al., 2021). Imperialism in Latin America and the Caribbean has been one of the greatest culprits in people being forced to flee their homelands and attempt to seek refuge in the U.S.A. When communities arrive in the U.S.A., many face poverty, racism, xenophobia, and lack of access to basic needs. Lack of resources and attempts at survival, like assimilation and acculturation, increase the likelihood of mental health complications (Farrell, 2022; Hyman & Dussault, 2000; Mengistu & Manolova, 2019). Acculturation is the process of learning and adopting characteristics of the dominant culture, while assimilation refers to integrating the dominant culture while disconnecting from one's culture of origin. Poverty disproportionately impacts communities of Color (Farrigan, 2021). Research is almost nonexistent regarding the experiences of perinatal individuals who are not part of dominant communities, such as Indigenous peoples, transgender parents, and caregivers with intellectual and developmental disabilities, among many others (Akobirshoev et al., 2019; Carone et al., 2021; Heck, 2021). The lack of research directly impacts the development of culturally appropriate screening and interventions. Critical assessment of systemic and interpersonal power dynamics can support providers in avoiding harmful discourses like "treatment resistance." When we see a community with low engagement numbers or hesitation to seek support, we must reflect on the conditions that have created and maintained those outcomes. Reflection helps us avoid placing the blame on clients rather than on the barriers created by an unjust system.

PROVIDER STANCE

An anti-oppressive lens in the perinatal period can help providers explore how different systems interact with individuals and impact well-being. Understanding risk involves focusing on barriers and collaborating with communities towards equity, liberation, and belonging. Community collaboration is essential in developing and integrating effective treatment and assessment strategies. Providers can partner with clients to explore what it is like for them to seek support. This action might ask questions throughout treatment, like, *"What was it like for you to come here today? When you think about our work together, I wonder if you feel heard, seen, or validated. What can I do to be a better listener or collaborator?"* Providers might find giving some information or rationale for asking these questions helpful. For instance, I might tell a client, *"I know that seeking help is scary, and people are often concerned about what it means to meet with a mental health provider. How is being here with me for you?"* Providing a rationale for why we ask questions is a tool for balancing the power dynamics by highlighting transparency. The explanation helps us to think about the purpose of our questions and to share that with the client. It is equally vital for these questions to continue throughout the therapeutic relationship.

I encourage clinicians to approach screening perinatal individuals with cultural humility and curiosity (See Chapter 7 for more on assessment). Humility reminds us that we do not have all the answers, and curiosity helps us partner with the person. A slew of clinically validated tools is available with a quick internet search, some for free and others for a fee. I will critically discuss some standard tools. My goal is that you approach talking about PMH conditions from the understanding that people are the experts in themselves. The tools can serve as a guide or aid to our collaboration. As clinicians, we have some knowledge and skills to support families. At the same time, we must remain vigilant that our clinical lens often intersects with systems of oppression, implicit biases, and ethnocentrism. Most screening tools, even when validated, require a critical lens, especially when working with individuals of the global majority. After all, the construct of psychopathology arises from the belief that some behavior is typical, while that which is not is problematic. AOT considers all inequalities in power dynamics as harmful. For clinicians, this means that the therapeutic relationship always has the potential to create unintentional harm. A lack of curiosity can push us to over-pathologize or miss significant concerns. Most of us humans struggle with recognizing when we need help. We often push ourselves to the edge and reach for help once we are out of emotional bandwidth. Caregivers and families from historically marginalized communities have the added complexity that asking for help has led to and, in many instances, continues to lead to harm. Not recognizing this truth will lead to further marginalization within and potentially beyond the clinical relationship.

Some caregivers might come into our practices because they struggle with a PMH condition. They might have been in therapy in the past, done research on how they are feeling, and are ready to discuss diagnosis and treatment. Many other caregivers might not know or understand that what they are experiencing might result from emotional distress. The latter is especially true for child therapists, where the caregiver's mental health is not the focus of treatment. The parent may come in with concerns about their child and present significant anxiety or symptoms of posttraumatic stress. Therapists must use their clinical judgment to determine the level of readiness a caregiver might have to discuss the possibility of a PMH condition or complication. This caution does not mean that caregivers are fragile or cannot emotionally handle difficult conversations because this is untrue. It does mean that a failure to consider historical trauma, especially regarding the mental health system, can lead to harm. Mental health diagnoses are a reality in navigating the healthcare system. Some clinicians might be free to practice counseling without a clinical diagnosis, while those who accept insurance must often provide a diagnosis for service reimbursement. In cases where we must give a mental health diagnosis, it is crucial to clarify the meaning and purpose of diagnosing. For instance, we might explain that we must provide a diagnosis for insurance reimbursement. Therapists might find that reviewing the diagnostic criteria with the client can help make the process collaborative.

PMH CONDITIONS

The Marcé Society, a leading organization in the United Kingdom, is credited for establishing the field of perinatal mental health in the 1980s (Krohn & Meltzer-Brody, 2021). Since then, organizations like Postpartum Support International have helped create a community of providers that love and support perinatal people. The field of perinatal mental health recognizes six mental health conditions impacting pregnancy and postpartum: Depression, anxiety, OCD, trauma, bipolar disorder, and psychosis. The Diagnostic and Statistical Manual of Mental Disorders, Fifth Edition, Text Revision (DSM-5-TR™) does not include conditions specific to the perinatal period. Major Depression and Bipolar I and II Disorders include a peripartum onset specifier in the DSM-5-TR™, referring to the timeframe between pregnancy and four months postpartum. The perinatal field continues to advocate for having PMH complications or expanding current specifiers in future versions of the DSM (Davis et al., 2018). A lack of recognition presents an additional barrier to communities accessing care.

Below are six disorders recognized by the field, with common symptoms for each condition and a possible DSM-5 crossover.

Perinatal Depression

Possible DSM-5 diagnosis: Major Depressive Disorder; Adjustment Disorder with Depressed Mood

Presentation: Symptoms of depressive or adjustment disorder in addition to themes related to the baby, such as guilt, lack of interest, and, when severe, possible thoughts of harming self or baby. The person might experience distress, such as feeling like a terrible caregiver, disconnected from the baby, angry at loved ones, a sense of resentment, or different bodily concerns.

Perinatal Anxiety

Possible DSM-5 diagnosis: Adjustment Disorder with Anxious Mood; Panic Disorder

Presentation: Symptoms of anxiety and concerns about their capacity as a caregiver and the baby's well-being.

Perinatal Obsessive-Compulsive Disorder

Possible DSM-5 diagnosis: Obsessive Compulsive Disorder (OCD)

Presentation: Symptoms of OCD in addition to intrusive thoughts. Intrusive thoughts in the perinatal period can be scary to the individual and their loved ones. Ideas tend to be graphic and bizarre. The individual feels distressed about the thoughts and tries to do everything possible to avoid acting on them. Providers and loved ones might notice significant hypervigilance over the baby as evidenced by avoidance and fear of someone else caring for the baby or constantly checking that the baby is breathing.

Perinatal Trauma

Possible DSM-5 diagnosis: Acute Stress Disorder; Posttraumatic Stress Disorder

Presentation: Trauma responses might happen when exposed to rape, pregnancy complications, labor and delivery, or NICU stay.

Perinatal Bipolar Disorder

Possible DSM-5 diagnosis: Bipolar I Disorder I; Bipolar II Disorder

Presentation: Many individuals might experience the first manic or hypomanic episode postpartum. Clinicians working with clients experiencing depression collaborate to monitor any possible mood changes that may warrant further assessment or intervention. Monitoring is vital for people taking selective serotonin reuptake inhibitors (SSRIs) like Sertraline, as they are the most common psychotropic treatment for depression and contraindicated for Bipolar Disorder.

Postpartum Psychosis

Possible DSM-5 diagnosis: Brief Psychotic Episode; Bipolar Disorder I; Schizophrenia

Presentation: Psychosis can take place in the context of any of the diagnoses listed above. Postpartum psychosis is a rare condition impacting 1 to 2 out of every 1,000 births (Postpartum Support International, n.d.-a). The presentation includes a risk of suicidality and a slight chance of infanticide. As such, an episode of psychosis is a medical emergency requiring immediate care.

Please note that comorbidity of disorders is the norm regarding mental health complications, especially during the perinatal period. When talking to clients about diagnosis, I borrow the label perinatal distress from the work of Karen Kleiman. I use *distress* as an all-encompassing, neutral term for all mental health complications, even after the client and I have collaborated and agreed on a diagnosis.

SCREENING FOR PMH CONDITIONS

The Academy of Obstetrics and Gynecology (ACOG, 2018) recommends screening for PMH complications once during the perinatal period. Postpartum Support International (n.d.-b) recommends screening at least three times during pregnancy (first visit, second and third trimesters). They also recommend screening at the first postpartum visit and months three, six, nine, and twelve. Due to the impact of psychosocial stressors on emotional well-being, screening and assessment should be ongoing during the life of the treatment. A caregiver might experience mild distress in the third month and significant complications at a later visit. The continuing relationship between stressors and well-being suggests the need for continuous assessment. Clinicians can collaborate with clients throughout treatment to determine changes in presentation and areas that need further attention. Therapists may observe that as they foster trust and the clinical relationship deepens, the client might share new concerns that will impact our understanding of the present problem. As we approach screening, we must consider the nature and quality of the client–therapist relationship:

- What identities are present?
- How are we, as clinicians, addressing power imbalances?
- What is the quality of the relationship?
- What are the individual, community, and ancestral experiences with the healthcare system and other power organizations like Child Protective Services?

I find in my practice that regardless of whether there is a perinatal condition present or not, caregivers experience feelings of shame and guilt constantly. Not only do caregivers worry, *"Am I good enough?" "Can I protect my child?"* but they tend to be one of the groups that receive the most unsolicited advice, reinforcing the belief that there is one right way of caregiving. We will talk about reflective practice in Chapter 5, but I want to mention here that we must constantly reflect on the impact of our words, actions, and message delivery during all stages of client care. As noted in Tenet 1, an anti-oppressive lens entails engagement in constant self-awareness (Tenets Initiative, 2018).

Here are some considerations for framing the screening of PMH complications:

- **Explore the person's understanding of what they are experiencing**. We want to know from their lens what their thoughts, behaviors, and emotions mean. Understanding the client's meaning can help providers correct dominant interpretations. Questions like, *"How has it been for you emotionally to be a caregiver?"* or *"How are you really feeling?"* can yield meaningful information regarding the person's inner world.
- **Normalize the difficulties of the transition to caregiverhood and caring for young children**. It can be hard to normalize concerns that impact life. I lean towards the statement, *"Feeling terrible is common, and yet we still don't talk about it or hear about it enough."* Providers must exercise caution to avoid disregarding the reality the person is experiencing when naming the societal push to be a perfect caregiver. Caring for a young child is difficult, even without mental health complications. Most caregivers are not living their best lives at two, three, and even five months

postpartum. Bodies, relationships, daily tasks, and identity change in each perinatal period. Change is hard, but losing a sense of yourself while providing for your child can be unbearable.

- **Provide psychoeducation on PMH complications, their frequency, and how often they are overlooked**. The slew of changes when a baby joins a family makes this period highly vulnerable. At the same time, because society does not talk about these changes, the experience is almost invisible. It is hard for humans to hear pain and for there to be nothing we can do to stop it. Many might make an "at least" statement when we hear the pain. Here is a typical example:

  Birthing person: I thought I was going to die. The pain was unbearable; I was vomiting on myself, and no one was listening to me.
  Listener: Oh, my goodness! *At least* your baby was healthy.

- **Use the "one drop and explore" guideline**. Share small amounts of information and check with the client how it feels for them. I learned the drop and explore tool from my training in a model named Facilitating Attuned Interactions (FAN). The FAN is a reflective approach to working with families that helps providers attune to the person's needs (Heller & Breuer, 2015). You can read more about this model in Chapter 5. Here is an example of drop and explore: "*Postpartum depression is extremely common. Some people might feel not quite like themselves, while others might feel ashamed and guilty for how horrible they are feeling. I wonder what it has been like for you?*"

- **If you have lived experience or learned how challenging struggling is from other caregivers, share it with clients**. My advanced training in psychotherapy taught me not to share anything personal in counseling. I remember creating a script for responding when clients asked personal questions. However, this way of relating does not work for me at this time in my life, nor does it support balancing power dynamics in the clinical relationship. I invite you to explore what aspects of self-disclosure are clinically appropriate for you through an anti-oppressive lens. No one can answer this for you; there is no one-step guide to being an anti-oppressive practitioner. However, the idea of the therapist as a blank slate that shares nothing does not honor a sense of community and authenticity central to many people from the global majority.

- **Screen all caregivers at treatment onset, pregnancy, and when a new baby/toddler joins the family**. You can explain to caregivers that screening is provided to all new clients and growing families. Making emotional wellness screening a regular part of treatment is vital for providers focusing on the dyadic relationship or those who only work with the child. Conditions can develop at any point in the perinatal period. Continuous screening is vital because people need time to establish trust in a relationship.

- **Consider the relationship between intersectionality and social determinants of health (SDH)**. SDH is a term that describes non-medical influences on health outcomes (Braveman et al., 2011). The U.S. Department of Health and Human Services (n.d.) defines SDH as "the conditions in the environments where people are born, live, learn, work, play, worship, and age that affect a wide range of health, functioning, and quality-of-life outcomes and risks" (para. 1). SDH can provide an intersectional lens where clinicians can explore the impact of structural racism, transgenerational trauma, and systemic barriers on the lives of perinatal individuals and their children. A systemic lens can support providers in recognizing how different SDHs can impact well-being. This step can help providers avoid discourses and interventions that blame the individual for outcomes (Matthews et al., 2021).
- **Explore risk factors**. Different life challenges can create risk for mental health complications in the perinatal period. When psychosocial stressors compound, wellness takes a back seat as our nervous systems go into survival mode. Figure 3.1 includes a list of common risk factors. Please share this list with clients as you consider the possibility of complications. Many individuals come into counseling experiencing various situations that affect their well-being. What can look like depression might result from a violent relationship and lack of support. Awareness of the multiple factors impacting function is vital to accurate diagnosis and lowering instances of over-pathologizing.

SCREENING TOOLS

Note that no validated tool will substitute the need for establishing a trusting relationship with a culturally attuned provider. Your clinical interview is the most powerful tool for assessing whether a complication is present. Providers using validated screening tools must partner with families to gather somatic and cognitive information regarding symptom presentation. For an in-depth understanding of conducting a clinical assessment for perinatal individuals, please check out Chapter 7.

Validated tools are helpful resources for screening mental health conditions. I will briefly describe three standard screening tools to find a balanced middle ground between AOT and the systems clinicians interact with, such as funders and payees. I will preface this section by reminding practitioners that even when we rely on standardized tools, a relational approach to delivery is critical to building

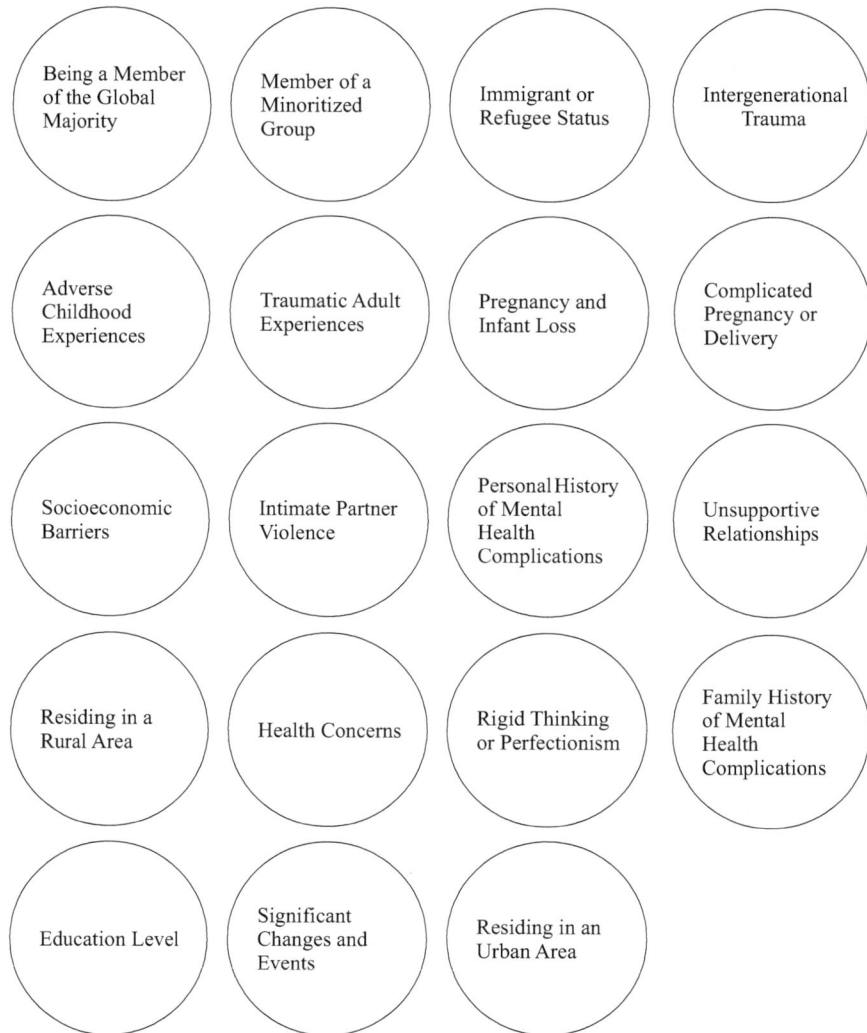

FIGURE 3.1 Risk Factors in the Perinatal Period

a trusting relationship where people might be more likely to seek support. No tool can fully assess individuals' specific needs and presentations from all cultural backgrounds. Conversations, further exploration, and collaboration are necessary to understand the client's concern. When screening tools are provided to clients to fill alone in the lobby or between sessions, we must ensure that we take precautions to discuss how disconnected it can feel to receive this form and how scary the questions can be to many.

The *Edinburgh Postnatal Depression Scale* (EPDS) is a ten-item self-report measure and one of the most commonly used screening tools. The EPDS screens for depression, anxiety, and suicidality. Several studies revealed that further testing is needed to strengthen the questionnaire's cross-cultural validity (Chan et al., 2021; McBride et al., 2014; Shrestha et al., 2016; Zubaran et al., 2010). Specifically, concerns regarding the validity of the EPDS include significantly lower detection of depression among non-Western groups like Indigenous populations and immigrants.

The *Patient Health Questionnaire-9* (PHQ-9) is a nine-question self-report measure for depression. The instrument is a viable option for screening depression during the perinatal period and has strong cross-cultural validation among some diverse groups (Harry et al., 2021; Wang et al., 2021). Importantly, Harry et al. (2021) found that the PHQ-9 might not fully capture depression among Alaska Native and American Indian populations. The researchers explained that the vast cultural diversity among Indigenous communities must be accounted for in the validation process of cross-cultural tools.

The *Generalized Anxiety Disorder-7* (GAD-7) is a self-report measure for anxiety comprising seven questions. The GAD-7 can be a helpful tool for screening anxiety but is not validated for the perinatal period (Mazzoni et al., 2021; Simpson et al., 2014). A 2015 study on cultural biases in the GAD-7 revealed the possibility of the tool underrepresenting the severity of anxiety symptoms among Black/African American populations (Parkerson et al., 2015). The GAD-7 is a commonly used tool for screening anxiety. Although useful, it must be accompanied by a comprehensive and culturally attuned assessment (See Chapter 7).

Zubaran et al. (2010) explained, "The significant variation in the prevalence figures of PPD according to studies conducted in different non-Western countries suggests that the way PPD presents itself cannot be matched transculturally by a stationary diagnostic criteria established according to Western yardsticks" (p. 361). There is no perfect tool to screen all people. Perhaps the sweet spot is to create space to hear and honor the client's lived expertise, including their understanding of what they are experiencing.

DISCUSSING CONCERNS WITH THE CLIENT

Mental health complications are complex. Biological and environmental vulnerabilities can compound during the perinatal period, leading to a higher risk for severity and comorbidity. During my years in practice, I have worked with clients who experience a sense of relief when I share a diagnosis and others who do not. Individuals have told me that knowing what they are experiencing has a name makes them feel relieved and that their experience is real. However, as we will continue to discuss in this book, diagnostic labels have been weaponized against communities facing marginalization. Individuals who lived in the foster-care system might have experienced parallel realities where trauma was overlooked, and a stigmatizing diagnosis might have been given. I encourage providers to be mindful when talking about possible diagnoses with clients. Through a trauma-informed lens, we can accept that diagnostic labels have been historically harmful and approach our work as such.

Providers might find it helpful to inquire about the client's and their ancestor's experience with diagnosis and the mental health system. An inquiry into this type of history can help the individual know that the therapist has some awareness of harm and is invested in the client's well-being. Suppose therapists work directly with insurance or another system requiring a diagnosis for treatment reimbursement. In that case, therapists must hold this conversation with clients sooner rather than later. Diagnosis might be beneficial even in cases where we are not seeking insurance reimbursement, as, when attuned to the client's needs, diagnosis can guide treatment and support progress. However, how we utilize and communicate the diagnosis to the client must meet the person's cultural needs and align with an AOT model.

Depending on the needs of the individual, the provider might find that the client would like to engage their loved ones in their care. I inform clients at intake that they can invite loved ones into our sessions. Therapists will learn about important people in the client's life and possible concerns. These moments represent ports of entry for reminding the client that their loved one is welcome to join a session to learn more about how to support them. During sessions with loved ones, the term *perinatal* or *postpartum distress* is a relatable way to explain what the individual is experiencing. There might be times when, due to cultural reasons, dynamics, or schedules, the client's loved one might not be able or willing to attend a session. Therapists can then partner with clients to think about ways to obtain support. These include problem-solving with clients in ways they want to share concerns and meet their needs. The client must lead with their ideas, as how they communicate might differ from how the provider has been trained to provide support. For example, setting boundaries can look different in families within the dominant American culture than in Black and Brown families. While it might be appropriate in some Westernized communities to use a direct and assertive communication style to tell an older family member, "*I would like to hold my boundaries and stop this conversation as it is unsupportive of my mental health*," this communication style may not be attuned within a Latin Caribbean immigrant family. Providing attuned support will depend on the specifics of each family.

CASE EXAMPLE

Sabrina, pronouns they/them, is a 33-year-old Cuban individual experiencing depression following the birth of their baby four months ago. Sabrina was referred to counseling with me after a visit with the OBGYN, where they reported not sleeping, low appetite, and irritability.

In the first session, they reported feeling hopeless and guilty about their role as a parent.

Sabrina became visibly distressed as they stated, *"I am not made for this. I thought I would be able to cope, but I feel lost."* I provided validation by discussing the difficulties of caring for a young child with limited support and the societal expectation that people with uteruses have a superhuman ability to be a parent. We discussed the messages Sabrina received about what the postpartum period would be like and their transition to parenthood. Sabrina reported feeling increasingly better during the second and third sessions, stating, *"These sessions are really helping me."* Being seen and heard can heal our souls. However, two to three sessions are generally insufficient to make impactful change. As a Latina, I wondered about the need to "ser fuerte" (be strong) in our Latino communities and explored this gently with the client. The discourse of mothers (and women) needing to present a strong front in the face of adversity is prevalent in many Black and Brown communities. I explored the idea with Sabrina.

Therapist: We have to put on the "ser fuerte" armor each morning. Sometimes, it feels like there is no choice, as others expect us to handle everything like before.
Sabrina: I have no choice but to push forward.
Therapist: I wonder if there could be a way to put the armor aside for a little bit of time while we are together.
Sabrina: I don't know how to do that.
Therapist: It's a hard ask. We can take it one step at a time. One idea is to look at what you might be experiencing right now.

I introduced the PHQ-9 by explaining to Sabrina that this was a way to explore possible concerns. Instead of beginning from the first question, I started with question number six, "Feeling bad about yourself —or that you are a failure or have let yourself or your family down" (Kroenke et al., 1999, para. 6). When I asked the question, Sabrina became tearful and shared feelings like they were letting their family down.

Sabrina: I am failing my family. They need me to be strong and available, but I am tired and sad. I don't want them to see me like this.
Therapist: It's hard to show up as ourselves when people are used to seeing our strong side.
Sabrina: Well, you know, al mal tiempo buena cara (loosely translated as: When times get tough, put on a good face).
Therapist: That's a lot of work.

Sabrina: I can't even do it well anymore. I am not eating or showering.
Therapist: Thank you for sharing that. That is putting the armor aside.

This conversation became the entry point for deepening the clinical relationship and entering treatment. We used the PHQ-9 as a port of entry to a conversation rather than a diagnostic tool. There was something about seeing the statement written down that helped Sabrina to know they were not alone.

SUMMARY

PMH complications must be understood in the context of intersectionality and systemic pressures. Historical and present-day trauma impacts birthing people's capacity to access mental health services. Applying an anti-oppressive lens to screening PMH complications includes understanding the root of medical mistrust. Providers are encouraged to continuously screen for complications and stressors when working with perinatal individuals. The EPDS, PHQ-9, and GAD-7 are standard measures for anxiety and depression. Because of concerns with cross-cultural validity, screening with a tool requires engagement in a collaborative, culturally attuned relationship.

REFERENCES

Academy of Obstetrics and Gynecology. (2018). Patient screening. https://www.acog.org/programs/perinatal-mental-health/patient-screening

Akobirshoev, I., Mitra, M., Parish, S. L., Moore Simas, T. A., Dembo, R., & Ncube, C. N. (2019). Racial and ethnic disparities in birth outcomes and labour and delivery-related charges among women with intellectual and developmental disabilities. *Journal of Intellectual Disability Research*, *63*(4), 313–326. https://doi.org/10.1111/jir.12577

Braveman, P., Egerter, S., & Williams, D. R. (2011). The social determinants of health: Coming of age. *Annual Review of Public Health*, *32*(1), 381–398. https://doi.org/10.1146/annurev-publhealth-031210-101218

Carney, C. J. J. (2021, January 4). The role of experimentation and medical mistrust in COVID-19 skepticism. *The Elm*. University of Maryland. https://elm.umaryland.edu/voices-and-opinions/Voices--Opinions-Content/The-Role-of-Experimentation-and-Medical-Mistrust-in-COVID-19-Vaccine-Skepticism-.php

Carone, N., Rothblum, E. D., Bos, H. M. W., Gartrell, N. K., & Herman, J. L. (2021). Demographics and health outcomes in a U.S. probability sample of transgender parents. *Journal of Family Psychology*, *35*(1), 57–68. https://doi.org/10.1037/fam0000776

Chan, A. W., Reid, C., Skeffington, P., & Marriott, R. (2021). A systematic review of EPDS cultural suitability with Indigenous mothers: A global perspective. *Archives of Women's Mental Health*, *24*, 353–365. https://doi.org/10.1007/s00737-020-01084-2

Davis, W. N., Raines, C., Indman, P., Meyer, B. G., & Smith, A. (2018). History and purpose of postpartum support international. *Journal of Obstetric, Gynecologic & Neonatal Nursing*, *47*(1), 75–83. https://doi.org/10.1016/j.jogn.2017.10.004

Farrell, M. V. (2022). Restoring birth as ceremony can promote health equity. *AMA Journal of Ethics*, *24*(4), 326–332. https://doi.org/10.1001/amajethics.2022.326

Farrigan, T. (2021, August 9). Rural poverty has distinct and racial patterns. Economic Research Service. https://www.ers.usda.gov/amber-waves/2021/august/rural-poverty-has-distinct-regional-and-racial-patterns/

First Nations Health Authority & Office of the Provincial Health Officer. (2021). Sacred and strong: Upholding our matriarchal roles. https://www.fnha.ca/Documents/FNHA-PHO-Sacred-and-Strong.pdf

Harry, M. L., Coley, R. Y., Waring, S. C., & Simon, G. E. (2021). Evaluating the cross-cultural measurement invariance of the PHQ-9 between American Indian/Alaska Native adults and diverse racial and ethnic groups. *Journal of Affective Disorders Reports*, *4*, 100121. https://doi.org/10.1016/j.jadr.2021.100121

Heck, J. L. (2021). Postpartum depression in American Indian/Alaska Native women: A scoping review. *The American Journal of Maternal/Child Nursing*, *46*(1), 6–13. https://doi.org/10.1097/NMC.0000000000000671

Heller, S. S., & Breuer, A. (2015). Fussy baby network New Orleans and Gulf Coast: Using the FAN to support families. *Zero To Three Journal*, *35*(3), 56–62.

Hyman, I., & Dussault, G. (2000). Negative consequences of acculturation on health behaviour, social support and stress among pregnant Southeast Asian immigrant women in Montreal: An exploratory study. *Canadian Journal of Public Health*, *91*(5), 357–360. https://doi.org/10.1007/bf03404807

Kroenke, K., Spitzer, R. L., & Williams, J. B. W. (1999). Patient Health Questionnaire-9 (PHQ-9) [Database record]. APA PsycTests. https://doi.org/10.1037/t06165-000

Krohn, H., & Meltzer-Brody, S. (2021). The history of perinatal psychiatry. In E. Cox (Ed.)., *Women's mood disorders: A clinician's guide to perinatal psychiatry*. Springer. https://doi.org/10.1007/978-3-030-71497-0_1

Matthews, K., Morgan, I., Davis, K., Estriplet, T., Perez, S., & Crear-Perry, J. A. (2021). Pathways to equitable and anti-racist maternal mental health care: Insights from Black women stakeholders. *Health Affairs*, *40*(10), 1597–1604. https://doi.org/10.1377/hlthaff.2021.00808

Mazzoni, S. E., Bott, N. L., & Hoffman, M. C. (2021). Screening for perinatal anxiety. *American Journal of Obstetrics and Gynecology*, *224*(6), 628–629. doi:https://doi.org/10.1016/j.ajog.2021.03.00

McBride, H. L., Wiens, R. M., McDonald, M. J., Cox, D. W., & Chan, E. K. H. (2014). The Edinburgh Postnatal Depression Scale (EPDS): A review of the reported validity evidence. In B. D. Zumbo & E. K. H. Chan (Eds.), *Validity and validation in social, behavioral, and health sciences* (pp. 157–174). Springer International Publishing/Springer Nature. https://doi.org/10.1007/978-3-319-07794-9_9

Mengistu, B. S., & Manolova, G. (2019). Acculturation and mental health among adult forced migrants: A meta-narrative systematic review protocol. *Systematic Reviews*, *8*(184). https://doi.org/10.1186/s13643-019-1103-8

National Partnership for Women & Children. (2020). Past as present: America's sordid history of medical reproductive abuse and experimentation. https://www.nationalpartnership.org/our-work/resources/health-care/past-as-present-americas-sordid-history-of-medical-reproductive-abuse-and-experimentation.pdf

Owens, D. C., & Fett, S. M. (2019). Black maternal and infant health: Historical legacies of slavery. *American Journal of Public Health*, *109*(10), 1342–1345. https://doi.org/10.2105/AJPH.2019.305243

Parkerson, H. A., Thibodeau, M. A., Brandt, C. P., Zvolensky, M. J., & Asmundson, G. J. G. (2015). Cultural-based biases of the GAD-7. *Journal of Anxiety Disorders*, *31*, 38–42. https://doi.org/10.1016/j.janxdis.2015.01.005

Postpartum Support International. (n.d.-a). Postpartum Psychosis. https://www.postpartum.net/learn-more/postpartum-psychosis/

Postpartum Support International. (n.d.-b). Screening recommendations. https://www.postpartum.net/professionals/screening/

Rodriguez, R., & Garcia, M. A. (2013). First, do no harm: The U.S. sexually transmitted disease experiment in Guatemala. *American Journal of Public Health*, *103*(12), 2122–2126. https://doi.org/10.2105/AJPH.2013.301520

Shrestha, S. D., Pradhan, R., Tran, T. D., Gualano, R. C., & Fisher, J. R. R. W. (2016). Reliability and validity of the Edinburgh Postnatal Depression Scale (EPDS) for detecting perinatal common mental disorders (PCMDs) among women in low- and lower-middle-income countries: A systematic review. *BMC Pregnancy Childbirth*, *16*(72), 1–19. https://doi.org/10.1186/s12884-016-0859-2

Simpson, W., Glazer, M., Michalski, N., Steiner, M., & Frey, B. N. (2014). Comparative efficacy of the Generalized Anxiety Disorder 7-item scale and the Edinburgh Postnatal Depression Scale as screening tools for Generalized Anxiety Disorder in pregnancy and the postpartum period. *The Canadian Journal of Psychiatry*, *59*(8), 434–440. https://doi.org/10.1177/070674371405900806

Smithsonian. (n.d.). The historical significance of doulas and midwives. https://nmaahc.si.edu/explore/stories/historical-significance-doulas-and-midwives

Tenets Initiative. (2018). Diversity-informed tenets for work with infants, children & families/Principios informados en la diversidad para trabajar con bebés, niños, niñas y familias. Irving Harris Foundation. https://diversityinformedtenets.org/download-the-tenets/

U.S. Department of Health and Human Services. (n.d.) Social determinants of health. https://health.gov/healthypeople/priority-areas/social-determinants-health

Wang, L., Kroenke, K., Stump, T. E., & Monahan, P. O. (2021). Screening for perinatal depression with the Patient Health Questionnaire depression scale (PHQ-9): A systematic review and meta-analysis. *General Hospital Psychiatry*, *68*, 74–82. https://doi.org/10.1016/j.genhosppsych.2020.12.007

Zubaran, C., Schumacher, M., Roxo, M., & Foresti, K. (2010). Screening tools for postpartum depression: Validity and cultural dimensions. *African Journal of Psychiatry*, *13*(5), 357–365. https://doi.org/10.4314/ajpsy.v13i5.63101

CHAPTER FOUR

Supporting Babies and Young Children

Picture a small child in your mind's eye. Sit with that image briefly as you think about what you notice. How does the child look? Are they smiling, sleeping, or playing? What surrounds them? Who is in their lives? What is available to them? What is their experience of the world, others, and themselves like? What is important to them? Who sees them? How do you understand their experience? Who makes them feel safe? We can continue with questions and reflections as we try to capture their felt experience. Acknowledging the child's experience is vital to bringing their voice into the therapeutic space. When we connect with their experience, we can honor their humanity and the different roles and relationships they carry. Children are worthy of being seen and heard. They are people with feelings and emotions. We live in a society that does not honor children. The lack of attention to the specific needs of children, especially young ones, has detrimental rippling costs across generations (Zero to Three, 2017). This chapter grounds our understanding of the mental well-being of young children from a historical and present-day lens.

THE BEGINNINGS OF THE CHILD WELFARE SYSTEM

As you consider tools to support the well-being of babies and young children, I encourage you to note how the past informs the present. We must understand history to conceptualize a framework that includes children. I grew up in a community where we often said, "*Borron y cuenta nueva*" (loosely translated as "Forget the past and start over"). That narrative arises as a protection from feelings of powerlessness in the face of intergenerational exploitation and trauma.

DOI: 10.4324/9781003286394-6

If we think about dissociating from past experiences as a survival mechanism, we can re-associate or reconnect with our story in times of healing. I hope we come from a place of healing and liberation each time we work with a family. Counseling from an anti-oppressive lens requires intentional reconnection with history, as building a structure without examining its foundation is dangerous. The Tenet, "Self-awareness leads to better services for families," reinforces the importance of knowing the impact of systems of oppression on the lives of children and families (Tenets Initiative, 2018, para. 1). It also calls for providers to recognize how oppression shapes our thinking, interventions, and in this case, how we support children. A lack of examination of the past can lead us to create on quicksand instead of solid ground. When we do not examine the foundation that we are building upon, we risk simple solutions to complex problems. Let us take the foster care system as an example. A child that experiences abuse and is removed from their caregiver and placed in the care of a foster family. Although it can seem like an idea that makes sense, what we know to be true is that children in foster care often experience a lack of stability through multiple temporary placements and retraumatization (Font & Gershoff, 2020).

Chapter 3 discussed some of the impacts of systemic oppression on the lives of perinatal people from historically marginalized backgrounds. The U.S. government's history of forcibly separating children from their families started with the kidnapping and trafficking of enslaved children during chattel slavery (Berry, 2018). Throughout history, the U.S.A. has "legally" separated African, Indigenous, Japanese, Chinese, and Latino children from their families (The Gathering for Justice, n.d.; Library of Congress, n.d.). Minoritized communities have experienced a range of deception and harm through the facade of establishing safety. In this section, you will have an opportunity to read and reflect on the impact of colonization and racism on the lives of children.

Attention to the needs of young children is a relatively new concept in our society. Even as the U.S.A. increased its attention to the protective rights of children regarding their safety, well-being, and development, abuse by systems of power continued. We see the start of a shift in children's rights in the late 1800s. However, as organizations and lawmakers increased their focus on children, this did not include Black or Indigenous children. Awareness of intergenerational experiences gives us a greater understanding of a child's ability to learn, feel, explore, and connect with others. New York was the first state to establish an organization to prevent child abuse in 1874 (Preibisch, 2022). In 1912, the U.S. government established the Federal Children's Bureau, known today as the Children's Bureau. Currently, each state is responsible for defining child abuse and neglect laws. The Children's Bureau sets minimum standards and administers funding for national child prevention programming with the support of the Child Abuse Prevention and Treatment Act (CAPTA) legislation enacted in 1974 (Child Welfare Information Gateway, n.d.; Children's Bureau, 2022). The CAPTA defines the minimum standards of abuse and neglect as "any recent act or failure to act on the part of a parent or caretaker, which results in death, serious physical or emotional harm, sexual abuse or exploitation …, or an act or failure to act which presents an imminent risk of serious harm" (CAPTAC, 2010, p. 24).

In the 1880s, the U.S.A. began kidnapping Indigenous children from their families and placing them in boarding schools to assimilate them into white culture and erase their Indigeneity (The National Native American Boarding School Healing Coalition, 2020). Children in boarding schools experienced genocide, abuse, and torture. As boarding schools waned, the Indian Adoption Project, which started in 1958, brought on another effort to remove children from their parents. Policies under this project enlisted social workers to coerce Indigenous families to give up their parental rights. U.S. authorities placed Indigenous children into non-Indigenous households, continuing the cycle of cultural genocide. Child Protective Services (CPS) had removed one in four Indigenous children from their families by the 1960s. Let that sink in, one in four. In 1978, through Indigenous advocacy, Congress passed the Indian Child Welfare Act (ICWA). The ICWA includes protections for Indigenous families during CPS involvement, like recognizing Tribal jurisdiction, encouraging kinship and Tribal placement, and protecting families from the coercive relinquishment of parental rights (Bureau of Indian Affairs, 2016). The ICWA is vital to supporting Indigenous culture and well-being and, in 2023, faced a potential overturn. An overturn might result in Tribes no longer having a say when CPS removes Indigenous children from their homes. Settler colonialism continues to threaten the lives of Indigenous families today.

Early schools in the nineteenth century were generally available to White males whose families were not living in poverty (Center on Education Policy, 2020). When girls were allowed to attend school, curriculums often differed from their male counterparts. Let us also remember that, until 1954, the law of the land upheld segregation in the school system under the auspices of the "separate but equal" doctrine (Legal Defense Fund, n.d.). *Brown vs. the Board of Education* changed some aspects of the U.S. educational system. However, it was not until 1960 that 6-year-old Ruby Bridges could attend a formerly all-white school in the South (Michals, 2015). Her attendance that year included daily escorting by federal marshals, hate demonstrations, and a class with no other students. In 2023, there are still more than 200 unresolved desegregation cases in the federal court system. (Legal Defense Fund, n.d.). For over 18 million children in the U.S.A. today, school access remains divided by race, ethnicity, or economic makeup due to the legacy of colonization, enslavement, and Jim Crow (U.S. Government Accountability Office, 2022). The legacy of slavery is present in the lives of Black and Brown families daily, leading to lower funding in schools and significant barriers to success than their White counterparts.

Let us look at another historical event as we understand the foundation of child well-being in the U.S.A. The Orphan Train Movement was a 75-year project ending in 1929 where charities kidnapped children from places in the East, like New York, and put them on a train to the West for farm labor or adoption (Trammell, 2009). Critics of the movement report that most families impacted by the Orphan Trains were European immigrants. It is essential to mention that immigrants from Italy, Greece, Poland, and many other places were not considered White in the late 1800s to early 1900s (Starkey, 2017). Charities placed children deemed homeless or abandoned in trains that moved across state lines without restriction (Trammell, 2009). People would then choose the children out of line-ups, most times for indentured servitude. There was no recordkeeping for most of the children as they would move from one station to the other in hope and fear of being chosen. The Orphan Trains separated children from their families and siblings, often forcing them to work, abusing, neglecting, and sometimes killing them. This movement is another piece of the foundational beginnings of our current child welfare system. Kidnapping and exploitation under the auspices of creating safety.

I lived in Miami, FL since we arrived in the U.S.A. in 1995. In 2019, I moved to the Pacific North West, and found stark differences in child abuse laws relating to domestic violence exposure. Having spent years working with children exposed to this kind of violence, seeing the difference was shocking. It was also a reminder of the lack of support that families experience all around. Even though exposure to domestic violence requires a mandated report in Florida, families and children still suffer due to oppressive systems and their lack of appropriate support. Lack of proper support creates harm. Miller and Burch (2014) published *Innocents Loss* in the *Miami Herald* newspaper. *Innocents Loss* is a six-year investigative report on 534 children who died due to abuse and neglect while having Child Protective Services involvement. Although child abuse and perinatal mental health complications do not have a direct cause-and-effect relationship, the risk increases with the compounding of psychosocial stressors. There has to be a balance between removing children from their families and leaving families to fend for themselves in the face of systemic racism, colonization, capitalism, and all the other forms of oppression that can make it impossible to breathe. I am holding Tenet 2 in mind here, "Champion children's rights globally" (Tenets Initiative, 2018, para. 2). I do not know the answer, but current systems do not work. We need to keep the conversation going and take action with (not for) the communities we hope to support.

TAKING A MOMENT TO REFLECT

Let us consider these two basic systems for supporting family well-being: Child welfare and education.

- How does this history inform your understanding of the families you support?

  _____

  _____

  _____

- How do you imagine this history impacts families from historically marginalized communities?

  _____

  _____

  _____

- How can you "Work to acknowledge privilege and combat discrimination" (Tenet 3) in your work with babies, toddlers, and perinatal caregivers?

  _____

  _____

  _____

- How did ethnocentrism influence the decisions made during the examples given above?

  _____

  _____

  _____

- How do we see ethnocentrism impacting how we think about best practices for babies, young children, and their families?

  _____

  _____

  _____

We will bridge the development of the early relational field now that we have briefly looked at some historical components regarding children in the U.S.A.

INFANT AND EARLY CHILDHOOD MENTAL HEALTH (IECMH)

Zero to Three, a leading organization focused on babies and young children, defines IECMH as "the developing capacity of the child from birth to 5 years old to form close and secure adult and peer relationships; experience, manage, and express a full range of emotions; and explore the environment and learn—all in the context of family, community, and culture" (Zero to Three, 2017, p. 1). IECMH, or early relational health, is a multidisciplinary field encompassing all individuals and systems supporting children's well-being from prenatal to age 5, such as those in direct service industries and research and policy (Zeanah & Zeanah, 2019). However, the name IECMH is a constant topic of discussion among providers and advocates. There is something about having the word "mental health" in the title that makes it seem as though the field is reserved for mental health providers, alienating all who serve and care for children. When I tell people I specialize in infant mental health, I often get responses like, *"I've never heard of that,"* or *"How do you do that? Work with babies?,"* or simply the look of confusion on someone's face. The term "early relational health" makes sense to me. It aligns with my relational way of seeing the world and honors that babies are impacted by their relationships. Many providers that do not specialize in working with babies and young children are unfamiliar with the field and its relational approach. The myth that babies and young children do not understand their environment and are not impacted by changes also contributes to caregiver hesitancy to seek support when challenges present. Although children aged 0 to 5 are among the most vulnerable populations, early relational health is an emerging field (Zero to Three, n.d.).

Selma Fraiberg coined the term *infant mental health* in the 1970s (Brandt et al., 2014). Before this period, therapy models focused on infancy from the lens of its impact on adulthood rather than considering the caregiver–child relationship as a space for healing the baby and the adult. Fraiberg and colleagues developed infant–parent psychotherapy (IPP), one of the first early relationship treatment models. IPP focuses on bringing awareness to how the caregiver thinks about their child and how past experiences influence that relationship. This seminal work led to significant advancements in the mental health field for babies and young children. The field started seeing babies as beings with an emotional world worthy of attention and began researching ways to support young children. Intervention models in early relational health expanded with an increased focus on child development and the parent–child relationship. We want children to have the best chances of success as they navigate life. Today, various early relational health models reach families through three levels of support: Promotion, prevention, and intervention (Zero to Three, 2017).

Promotion approaches aim to support the general population. They might include resources that connect the community with parenting education, like apps, informational websites, free library programs, and activities that promote baby–caregiver bonding. Prevention strategies target risk and protective factors. Some examples include high-quality childcare and caregiver support groups. Each resource promotes community connection, child development, and caregiver respite. Interventions address underlying pathologies, such as mood and anxiety disorders and relational concerns between caregivers and their young children. These levels of support are vital to babies, young children, and families. However, they often only reach some community members while leaving out those with the most significant risk. Due to structural racism and the impact of colonization, communities of Color are less likely to have access to these services and supports. St. John (2019) explained that for the field to protect all children, it must advance social justice through an intersectional lens. Creating pathways for communities to lead in developing programming and goals is vital to imbuing liberatory approaches to the field.

DEVELOPMENT

Early childhood is an intricate time where development across socioemotional, cognitive, physical, and language domains moves exponentially quickly (Davies & Troy, 2020). Children can go from being unable to support their necks at birth to running around within about two years. Each child develops at their own pace. Development happens within the child's environment, including their relationships' quality and context. Understanding a child's well-being relies heavily on their developmental stage and capacities. Development occurs in an integrated fashion across domains as the child interacts with others (Zero to Three, 2016). For instance, social interactions can lead the way for language development and vice versa. Psychosocial stressors and access to resources can impact the developmental trajectory, placing children and families at risk.

Social interactions guide development by promoting exploration, expression of emotions, and curiosity (Brandt et al., 2014). Through the repetitive interactions a baby has with caregivers, the baby learns to be in the world and make sense of it. In relationships, the baby learns what to expect from others, including if they will meet their needs. Children are encouraged to explore when interactions with the environment and caregivers promote physical and emotional safety (Ray, 2015). Experiencing protection allows the baby to see new information as opportunities to experience the world. They explore their environment as they reach for their hands and feet, then toys, and eventually take steps towards and away from caregivers. While all this happens, babies learn how to relate to others through bids for connection by smiling, reaching, and turning their heads towards others. When safety and security are not present or consistent in a child's life, we might see limited exploration and connection with others. Consider the ripple effect of a child who experiences neglect, leading to a delay in meeting certain gross motor milestones. If caregivers do not give the child the appropriate support, fine motor development will also suffer, as large muscles develop before smaller ones. Over time, the child's socioemotional development might also slow. All domains can impact how the child navigates the world and how others see them. As the child enters pre-school, they might experience more frustration than other children due to the lack of support. Instructors and other caregivers might begin to see the child as problematic. Because the early childhood period is the foundation for life, if concerns go unaddressed or the child does not have an opportunity to catch up early, neglect can impact the course of adulthood.

Early relational health requires interdisciplinary collaboration. The collaboration should always entail the caregiver(s) and child at the forefront. We want to constantly understand what behaviors and concerns mean to caregivers. Partnership might also include coordination between the therapist and the childcare provider, speech and language pathologist, occupational therapist, home visitor, and any other support in that family's life. Collaborative care is challenging and crucial for effective services. It is difficult because it requires added work and time from support persons. It is essential, as each partner in the child's care is vital to understanding how to support the family. Children may present different behaviors in the context of relationships. For example, a child might have meal disruption with one caregiver and have no issues in their other household. Another consideration for building interdisciplinary collaboration is medical distrust. As mentioned in Chapter 3, medical distrust comes from past and present harm to historically marginalized communities. A lack of trust can also influence a family's capacity to ask for and receive support. Families often are not free to choose providers they would like to work with, as insurance, finances, transportation, the child welfare system, and other factors generally have the final say. This reality might help us consider how systems interacting might impact access and barriers for families. Implicit biases, lack of time, and limited training in the importance of relationships can impact interdisciplinary relationships among providers in different capacities where one provider may dismiss the work of the other.

The work with families in this early timeframe is preventative. Early support ensures we can connect with families before relationships suffer and concerns worsen. A developmental screener can help us understand a piece of the picture of what the family is experiencing. One of the most common screening tools (and one that I use) is the Ages and States Questionnaire (ASQ-3), a self-report measure that caregivers can complete in less than 20 minutes, and its companion the ASQ-socioemotional scale (ASQ-SE-2) (Singh et al., 2017). Providers can access multiple screening tools to support families in understanding development and making appropriate referrals. A quick search online will yield numerous screening tools available for downloading. A challenge to appropriate screening, in addition to cultural relevance, is that many validated tools are available for purchase rather than for free download. Please use your clinical judgment when determining what developmental screeners to include in your practice. Remember that screening tools are not diagnostic tools nor a substitute for developing a collaborative relationship with the family (See Tenet 4). They help us dialogue with the family and determine whether further support from us or an outside provider is needed.

ADVERSE CHILDHOOD EXPERIENCES

In the 1990s, Kaiser Permanente and the Centers for Disease Control (CDC) explored risk factors contributing to disease and disability (Felitti et al., 1998). The study found a direct link between exposure to adverse childhood experiences (ACES) and the occurrence of disease and risk behaviors in adulthood. Most of the ACE study participants were White, middle-class, and with an average of 14.6 years of education. The study revealed that adversity is common, as over 50% of the study participants experienced at least one ACE. The ACES study helped understand the importance of the early childhood period. Today, many organizations provide families with an ACES questionnaire to help understand ongoing risk and best support methods. The ACES questionnaire is a ten-item scale developed from the 1998 study by Felitti and colleagues. The scale explores exposure to physical, emotional, and sexual abuse, neglect, and household dysfunction, such as parental substance abuse and incarceration.

Merrick et al. (2018) conducted a large-scale U.S. study between 2011 and 2014 to understand the intersection of ACES and demographic characteristics. The study spanned 23 states with over 200,000 participants. The findings revealed at least one ACE among 61% of respondents with higher exposure rates for Black and Hispanic individuals than their White counterparts. The results also showed higher rates for LGBTQ+ participants, individuals earning less than $15,000 annually, and people with less than a high school education. It is important to note that this study did not include any information on Indigenous communities. Sarche et al. (2017) explained that there needs to be more literature addressing the needs of Indigenous populations in the early childhood period. The authors posited that we could understand the risks associated with this period by examining some of the risk factors Indigenous communities experience in the U.S.A. Let us look at some of the statistics in the article related to Indigenous communities:

- Seventy percent of children live in poverty.
- Children are less likely to have a parent in favorable physical or emotional health.
- Children face stressors and violence at higher rates than do non-Indigenous children.

In 2012, the Philadelphia Research Committee expanded the ACE study to include the experience of urban communities with racial and socioeconomic diversity (Public Health Management Corporation, 2013). Their study led to a better understanding of community-level adversity. The Urban ACES includes the following four markers: Witnessing violence (separate from maternal domestic violence), discrimination, bullying, living in foster care, and adverse neighborhood experiences. I encourage providers who use the ACES questionnaire to also inquire about experiences related to Urban ACES to gather a comprehensive understanding of the family.

MENTAL HEALTH

There is also a lot of misinformation about the developmental needs and expectations of babies and young children. Little ones rely on the grown-ups and caregivers around them to protect them. When caregivers cannot access protective resources, their children risk experiencing harm. The myth that young children do not experience mental health complications leaves in isolation families needing support. It is hard for many of us to think about what depression might look like in a 3-year-old, let alone diagnose it. Still, children aged 0 to 5 can experience significant mental health complications (Zeanah & Zeanah, 2019). To diagnose a young child, one must distinguish typical behavior, culture, and developmental changes or regressions from psychiatric disorder symptoms. It is challenging to discern between developmentally and culturally expected behavior and concerns, as young children constantly change. Diagnosing is complicated.

Diagnosing young children has advantages and disadvantages. Under-and over-diagnosis of children of Color is a reality in our society. Caregivers might have concerns about what an evaluation or a possible label might mean to their child and how they are treated in school. Although mental health complications are common, they still hold a stigma in our society. At any given point, one in five individuals in the U.S.A. is experiencing a mental health condition (National Institute of Mental Health, 2021). Mental health complications are part of the human experience. Unfortunately, one of the main advantages of diagnosis comes from a systemic barrier. Diagnosis can lead to access to supportive services, as one is generally necessary for insurance reimbursement. The barrier in that scenario is that support is pathologized and often inaccessible. While some families can afford out-of-pocket payments, many cannot. Most providers cannot work without reimbursement for services, as most of us cannot access unlimited funds. Diagnosis for payment is a problematic cycle. Yet, we are navigating this system and must find ways to support and collaborate with families. Proper mental health screening can guide the course of treatment. It can help providers and families collaborate on the best way to support children. As the field is still emerging, diagnosing can also give us a common language to communicate with families and other providers. This issue is not one-sided. Providers can hold in mind the complexity of barriers and access to care as they navigate the system and partner families.

The *Diagnostic Classification of Mental Health and Developmental Disorders of Infancy and Early Childhood* (DC:0–5™) is a tool for guiding the diagnostic process of young children. I encourage providers to consider using the DC:0–5™ when diagnosing young children as part of the work. Check out Chapter 7 to read more about integrating the manual into conducting assessments. Clinicians can familiarize themselves by seeking training and supervision in this model.

CASE EXAMPLE

Much of the research in early childhood focuses on the impact of traumatic experiences on the developing brain. Not every traumatic experience a child has will become a trauma. However, compounding stressful situations or psychosocial stressors increases the risk of developmental and psychological complications (Zeanah & Zeanah, 2019). The longer the stressors exist in a child's and family's life without support, the more significant its impact. When we think about the well-being of babies and young children, we should also consider the caregivers in that child's life. Caregivers and their children are intricately connected; both suffer when one is not well. Let us look at a case example to help illustrate this reality.

Alex is a biracial, 28-year-old non-binary caregiver to Willow, their 15-month-old daughter. Alex has been residing at a shelter for the past six months and was reunified with Willow four months ago after a year-long separation following exposure to domestic violence. Alex reported that they had been in a violent relationship with Willow's father. Alex noted that Child Protective Services removed Willow following a domestic violence incident. Alex said that Willow has been crying inconsolably whenever sleep and feeding time begins. Alex worries that Willow is not getting enough nutrition, as the pediatrician reported concerns about her development, including weight.

Alex received a referral for infant mental health services and has worked with the provider for two months. During today's visit, Alex reports that they are 28 weeks pregnant. Alex does not share other details about the pregnancy but reports feeling shame and guilt at being unable to focus their entire energy on Willow. Alex notes that they had slept about two hours per night for the past few nights and experienced frequent panic attacks. They disclose that they also experienced similar symptoms when pregnant with Willow. Alex reports that during a particularly distressing panic attack last night, Willow began crying inconsolably and crawling towards the door. Alex reported that they did not know what to do and went into the bathroom to cry and not hear Willow cry.

Notice what comes up for you as you consider the details from this excerpt. Working with babies and young children can arouse intense feelings within us. Awareness of our internal world and experience as we sit with families is vital to our work. It honors the reflective process (See Chapter 5) and helps us engage Tenet 1, self-awareness (Tenets Initiative, 2018).

This case illustrates the compounding of psychosocial stressors caregivers might face. We see the impact of domestic violence, removal, reunification, homelessness, and parental mental health complications. Through a relational lens, we will explore multiple factors as we work with the family, including trauma, parental reflective functioning, parental stress, and Willow's developmental concerns.

Adding a systemic lens, we will consider ways to support the family with housing stability and encourage protection from future violence. The provider may discuss parent-only sessions to support the panic attacks while focusing on supporting the caregiver–child relationship at other meetings. Without careful attention and holding of the caregiver's experience, recommendations and discussions of Willow's well-being might be too difficult for Alex to bear. The clinician may notice this and gently follow their lead.

In cases where the provider misses the caregiver's needs, they may risk introducing interventions that can be experienced as harmful rather than helpful to the caregiver. For instance, focusing on relational health when panic attacks are unstable can increase caregiver stress, sending the unintentional message that they *should* be able to follow through. Since the baby was reunited with Alex four months ago, we might assume that there is continued CPS involvement.

I invite you to take a moment to reflect on the following questions:

- What might happen when other collaborators find out about the pregnancy?

  _____
  _____
  _____

- What will happen if Alex does not follow up on a separate referral for a mental health provider?

  _____
  _____
  _____

- What will the repercussions to Willow's psychological and physical well-being be without proper support?

  _____
  _____
  _____

- How might systemic trauma be impacting this family's experience?

  _____
  _____
  _____

- What else would you want to know as you partner with Alex and Willow?

  _____
  _____
  _____

Our brains have innate responses to fear and threat. When things become overwhelming, we can get ready to fight, flight, or freeze. Someone with a history of

CPS involvement is at risk of further complications, as their nervous system might be in a more vulnerable and reactive state. The systems we navigate tend to be punitive. If Alex fails to comply with a rule of the shelter, they might risk being kicked out, and if they do not listen to a provider's recommendation, they may lose custody of Willow. Alex's story is a painful reality for many families we support. As we consider the aspects of the story, I invite you to hold three concerns at the core of an anti-oppressive way of supporting families:

- Alex's well-being.
- Willow's well-being.
- Their relational well-being.

All three of these concerns are vital to allowing the full experience of all into the clinical space. We will explore specific skills to support the clinical relationship members in the assessment and treatment sections.

SUMMARY

Attention to the needs of babies and young children is relatively new in our society and in an emerging mental health field. Children aged 0 to 5 are among the most vulnerable populations in our society (Zero to Three, n.d.). The history of the child welfare system in the U.S.A. contains multiple narratives of kidnapping and exploitation of children. As providers consider supporting the needs of early childhood, they must understand how systemic racism and colonization impact our current systems of care. Psychosocial stressors and environmental changes affect the well-being of very young children. Children of these ages can experience the effects of trauma, mental health conditions, and developmental concerns. A relational and collaborative lens helps us partner with families to meet their children's individual and relationship needs.

REFERENCES

Berry, D. (2018, June 21). Breaking up families of Color, an American tradition as old as the slave trade. *Beacon Broadside*. https://www.beaconbroadside.com/broadside/2018/06/breaking-up-families-of-color-an-american-tradition-as-old-as-the-slave-trade.html

Brandt, K., Perry, B., Seligman, S., & Tronik, E. (2014). *Infant and early childhood mental health: Core concepts and clinical practice*. American Psychiatric Publishing.

Bureau of Indian Affairs. (2016). Final rule: Indian Child Welfare Act (ICWA). https://www.bia.gov/sites/default/files/dup/assets/bia/ois/raca/pdf/idc1-034295.pdf

Center on Education Policy. (2020). History and evolution of public education in the US. https://files.eric.ed.gov/fulltext/ED606970.pdf

Child Abuse Prevention and Treatment Act, 42 U.S.C. § 5101. (2010). https://www.congress.gov/111/plaws/publ320/PLAW-111publ320.pdf

Child Welfare Information Gateway. (n.d.). Definitions of child abuse and neglect. https://tinyurl.com/5dykd5ky

Children's Bureau. (2022, June 28). About. https://tinyurl.com/y4bm7xmw

Davies, D., & Troy, M. F. (2020). *Child development: A practitioner's guide*. Guildford Press.

Felitti, V. J., Anda, R. F., Nordenberg, D., Williamson, D. F., Spitz, A. M., Edwards, V., Koss, M. P., & Marks, J. S. (1998). Relationship of childhood abuse and household dysfunction to many of the leading causes of death in adults. The Adverse Childhood Experiences (ACE) Study. *American Journal of Preventive Medicine*, *14*(4), 245–258. https://doi.org/10.1016/s0749-3797(98)00017-8

Font, S. A., & Gershoff, E. T. (2020). Foster care: How we can, and should, do more for maltreated children. *Social Policy Report, (33)*3, 1–20. https://doi.org/10.1002/sop2.10

Legal Defense Fund. (n.d.). Brown V Board of Education: The case that changed America. https://www.naacpldf.org/brown-vs-board/

Library of Congress. (n.d.). Immigration and relocation in U.S. history. https://www.loc.gov/classroom-materials/immigration/

Merrick, M. T., Ford, D. C., Ports, K. A., & Guinn, A. S. (2018). Prevalence of adverse childhood experiences from the 2011–2014 behavioral risk factor surveillance system in 23 states. *JAMA Pediatrics*, *172*(11), 1038–1044. https://doi.org/10.1001/jamapediatrics.2018.2537

Michals, D. (2015). Ruby Bridges. https://www.womenshistory.org/education-resources/biographies/ruby-bridges

Miller, M. C., & Burch, A. D. S. (2014, March 16). 534 children who will never grow up. *Miami Herald*. https://media.miamiherald.com/static/media/projects/2014/innocents-lost/database/

National Institute of Mental Health. (2021). Mental illness. https://www.nimh.nih.gov/health/statistics/mental-illness

Preibisch, R. E. (2022). A history of child welfare in the United States. *MUsings: The Graduate Journal*. https://blogs.millersville.edu/musings/

Public Health Management Corporation. (2013). Findings from the Philadelphia urban ACES study survey. https://docs.google.com/forms/d/e/1FAIpQLSeMsb2FYIY20df8lOPhla2fvJvnZshSsXlspm7AA6q8AV3RYQ/viewform

Ray, D. (Ed.). (2015). *A therapist's guide to child development: The extraordinary normal years*. Routledge.

Sarche, M., Tafoya, G., Croy, C. D., & Hill, K. (2017). American Indian and Alaska Native boys: Early childhood risk and resilience amidst context and culture. *Infant Mental Health Journal*, *38*(1), 115–127. https://doi.org/10.1002/imhj.21613

Singh, A., Yeh, C. J., & Blanchard, B. S. (2017). Ages and stages questionnaire: A global screening scale. *Boletin Medical del Hospital Infantil de Mexico*, *74*(1), 5–12. http://dx.doi.org/10.1016/j.bmhimx.2016.07.008

Starkey, B. S. (2017). White immigrants weren't always considered white – and acceptable. https://andscape.com/features/white-immigrants-werent-always-considered-white-and-acceptable/

St. John, M. S. (2019). Reconceiving the field: Infant mental health, intersectionality, and reproductive justice. *Infant Ment Health Journal*, *40*(5), 608–623. https://doi.org/10.1002/imhj.21808

Tenets Initiative. (2018). Diversity-informed tenets for work with infants, children & families/Principios informados en la diversidad para trabajar con bebés, niños, niñas y familias. Irving Harris Foundation. https://diversityinformedtenets.org/download-the-tenets/

The Gathering for Justice. (n.d.). History of family separation. https://www.gatheringforjustice.org/familyseparation

The National Native American Boarding School Healing Coalition. (2020). Healing voices volume 1: Alaska Native boarding schools in the U.S. https://boardingschoolhealing.org/wp-content/uploads/2021/09/NABS-Newsletter-2020-7-1-spreads.pdf

Trammell, R. S. (2009). Orphan trains myths and legal reality. *The Modern American,* *(5)*2, 3–13. http://digitalcommons.wcl.american.edu/tma/vol5/iss2/3

U.S. Government Accountability Office. (2022, June 16). K-12 education: Student population has significantly diversified, but many schools remain divided along racial, ethnic, and economic lines. https://tinyurl.com/5n88n6zt

Zeanah, C. H., & Zeanah, P. S. (2019). Infant mental health: The clinical science of early experience. In C. H. Zeanah (Ed.), *The handbook of infant mental health* (4th edition, pp. 16–35). The Guilford Press.

Zero to Three. (2016). *DC:0–5™: Diagnostic classification of mental health and developmental disorders of infancy and early childhood*. Author.

Zero to Three. (2017). The basics of infant and early childhood mental health: A briefing paper. https://www.zerotothree.org/wp-content/uploads/2017/08/The-Basics-of-Infant-and-Early-Childhood-Mental-Health_-A-Briefing-Paper.pdf

Zero to Three. (n.d.). Safe babies. Transforming child welfare into the practice of strengthening child and family wellbeing. https://www.zerotothree.org/our-work/safebabies/

CHAPTER FIVE

Leaning into Reflective Practice

Consider a past or current relationship where you felt seen, heard, and accepted. Please bring it to mind and sit with that image for a few breaths, noticing the feelings and emotions that come up for you.

- What do you notice about the experience?

  _____
  _____
  _____

- What was it like to be seen and heard?

  _____
  _____
  _____

- How did you know that the other person was seeing and hearing you?

  _____
  _____
  _____

- What was it about them that allowed you to show up as yourself?

  _____
  _____
  _____

Reflection is a required ingredient for building and maintaining relationships. It moves us towards introspection in what we do and how we are (Pawl & St. John, 1998). In writing this book, I am attempting to connect with you. I think

DOI: 10.4324/9781003286394-7

about the impact of my communication on your experience moving through these pages. I am holding Tenet 6, "Understand that language can hurt or heal," as well as Tenet 1 and its call to self-awareness (Tenets Initiative, 2018). My words matter; how I share them with you will impact your journey. I wonder how you are experiencing me. What does the relationship feel like to you and me, even as we are separate in space and time? Through reflection, we can think about the impact of our actions and our way of being with others (Heller & Gilkerson, 2009). Reflective practice in mental health involves continuously exploring what it is like to be with the people we serve (Priddis & Rogers, 2017). This chapter explores the therapist's use of reflective practice to support connection and healing within the psychotherapeutic relationship.

THE THERAPEUTIC RELATIONSHIP

Let us start by engaging in reflection on our work. Please pause here and journal ideas, feelings, and thoughts regarding how you think about the therapeutic relationship.

- How do we think about the clinical relationship?

  _____
  _____
  _____

- How are we measuring its efficacy and strength?

  _____
  _____
  _____

- How do we think about the difference between what we do and how we are in session?

  _____
  _____
  _____

- What is the difference between implementing interventions and building a relationship?

  _____
  _____
  _____

- How do we know what the client's experience is?

  _____
  _____
  _____

- Do we have a space to reflect on what we imagine it is like to be the people we serve and how they might experience us?

  _____

  _____

  _____

Most clinicians recognize that the therapeutic relationship is the most critical component of effective counseling (DeAngelis, 2019). A relationship generally involves at least two people holding mutual trust and sharing a part of themselves. Sharing our story requires leaning into a sense of vulnerability where we expose parts of ourselves not generally shared with others. When one person leans in, it opens a gateway for the other to choose closeness or distance. They hold each other's stories as they choose proximity, deepening the relationship. Each member of a relationship brings a certain level of holding as we build trust. The therapist's role is to hold and contain the client's experience, but the client also holds on to a piece of us. We, too, are present and active in creating the space and its intimacy. Within the clinical relationship, the therapist holds the sharing of the other, generally with limited sharing of their personal story. The therapist's "leaning in" is different. However, vulnerability is still necessary to build trust. The client–therapist relationship contains closeness, but it differs from all other relationships one might experience. It is, in some ways, one-sided and, in others, collaborative. The power hierarchies are not balanced. When we look at it through this lens of one-sided holding, we can honor the vulnerability it takes for clients to share the most intimate parts of their lives with a provider. Can you also see the potential for harm here?

REFLECTION AND BELONGING

Reflection cannot happen without taking an anti-racist and anti-oppressive stance. Anti-oppressive theory (AOT) supports providers in balancing power dynamics, engaging in critical self-reflection, and responding to the needs of historically marginalized communities (Sakamoto & Pitner, 2005; Strier & Biyamin, 2014). The goal of anti-oppressive practices is to reduce harm and center the needs of vulnerable populations. Reflective practice entails an internal analysis of our client experiences. Reflection and anti-oppression are two ingredients that come together to welcome a partnership with the other. As you consider the questions below, notice how the identities present impact perceptions, feelings, and interactions.

- What is it like to be with this person?
- What is their life like?

- How is this person experiencing me?
- What did I notice within me when the client looked away, shifted in their seat, or seemed upset? What made me react in such a way?
- How did I choose the intervention?
- What did I notice about myself in my relationship with the other?

Through reflection, providers can explore what they do before, during, and after their work with clients (Bhola et al., 2022). Reflection before a session may entail thinking about how we feel and taking a few breaths to ground and connect with ourselves before meeting with the client. During the session, the therapist might maintain awareness of what they notice in their bodies, taking space to briefly see their inner world before intervening. The post-session reflection might include thinking, journaling, or discussing feelings and thoughts with a colleague. Our social positioning guides our reflection. It is the lens through which we see and experience the world. People have told me, *"Leave your problems at the door,"* meaning do not bring this part of your life into this space. I also remember trying to leave my problems at the door earlier in my work. I tried to shove pieces of me deeply into a container in my mind, onto a place where I could not access them. I imagine you might have found yourself trying to compartmentalize to survive so that others would not see that part of you. But how realistic is this? How is disconnection from ourselves conducive to a role where we must deeply connect with people's humanity?

In 1998, Pawl and St. John, pioneers in the early relational health field, published a transformational work titled "How you are is as important as what you do … in making a positive difference for infants, toddlers, and their families." If you work in the early relational health field, the phrase "how you are is as important as what you do" is familiar to you. It is a guiding principle of the work we do. The action we take with clients is essential, as is the stance and relationship we build. One does not work without the other. The authors outlined six principles for being and doing. Each principle is interconnected and helps us explore our work's humanity. The first is that all behavior has meaning. The meaning we give behavior depends on many factors. The assumptions we make in counseling impact the work and the relationship we are trying to build with the family. The second principle is that "everyone wants things to be better" (Pawl & St. John, 1998, p. 6). In this reflective stance, the therapist works to understand the motivations and goals of each family member. This idea serves as a reminder that everyone is trying to do their best with the resources they have. Third, we are providers and humans. How we are and what we do with families depends on our role, skills, and our full personhood, including culture and experience. Everything we are and do impacts how we view the world. Next, "don't just do something – stand there and pay attention" (p. 7) calls providers to observe before moving into action. The fifth principle is remembering that all we do is about building and maintaining relationships. Our work loses meaning without relationships. The last and one of my favorite principles is "do unto others as you will have others do unto others." All relationships impact each other. What we do, say, judge, and remain silent about connects to how we are and vice versa.

We are entering an era where people are encouraged to share and honor their experiences. As more organizations and systems recognize the dominant supremacy culture at play, the more its harm becomes visible. Silencing discomfort and the idea of professionalism are dominant discourses impacting how we relate to ourselves and to others. Now, because we are all swimming in white supremacy culture, none of us are immune. Those of us with close proximity to whiteness may have more freedom to honor our experiences than others. What happens when a provider misreads an interaction and misses an essential part of an individual's life? What determines that client's ability to revisit their concern? I wish I could say that the client will have many other opportunities to share their concern or that it is highly likely that the therapist will recognize the misattunement and work to repair the relationship. Psychotherapy can be a place of healing and, unfortunately sometimes, a place of harm. I learned from listening to Black colleagues that Black people often experience harm when counseling non-Black providers. A 2016 study revealed that over 80% of minoritized individuals had experienced at least one racial microaggression in counseling (Hook et al., 2016). Eighty percent is a pretty high number. I imagine that many of the therapists committing the microaggressions were well-meaning folk. Intentions matter, but they are not enough. We cannot repair that which is invisible to us. We need a guide and guidance into the unknown.

Reflective practice is a tool for navigating the unknown within the client–therapist relationship. We can practice reflection alone or in a relationship with other providers. As we hold other people's stories, providers must have a space to receive nurturing. Sometimes, the container for our story might be our time of meditation, journaling, or creating. Other times, it might be the stories we share with another who supports our work, such as a reflective supervisor or consultant. Several models for integrating reflective practice exist in the field. I am trained in and practice Facilitating Attuned Interactions (FAN). I bumped into FAN in 2012 while searching the internet for training on working with parents and babies. The training I found was called Fussy Baby and was led by the model's founder, Linda Gilkerson, and Anne Hogan. FAN is a component of Fussy Baby and has become a stand-alone framework for communication (Erikson Institute, 2015).

The FAN model helps providers reflect moment-to-moment as they sit with families (Gilkerson & Imberger, 2016). The goal of FAN is attunement to ourselves and to others. Gilkerson and Imberger (2016) explained that "Attunement in helping relationships is defined as feeling connected and understood" (p. 46). Attuning requires listening with our eyes, ears, and heart to ensure that our presence connects, responds, and provides what the client needs moment to moment. Connecting to what the other is feeling requires curiosity. Curiosity helps us remember that we do not have the answers and that we might make mistakes in our effort to connect. Attunement can guide repair and reconnection when our responses do not connect and reflect understanding of the client.

The model reflects a way of being that connects us with our internal world and helps us question how the people we support might feel. The FAN model has five processes: calming (mindful self-regulation), feeling (empathic inquiry), thinking (collaborative exploration), doing (capacity building), and reflecting (integration). The calming process reminds us to be attuned to our internal world before, during, and after each session. When strong feelings come up for us and others in a session, providers can lean into tools such as a deep breath to help bring the clarity and focus required to attune to the family's needs. Calming our inner world can help us know if the caregiver needs more space to explore and validate *feelings*, to *think* together about options, to *do* and try out new skills, or to *reflect* on what they know. If you are familiar with FAN, you will also recognize its impact on my life and work as you read this text.

We will continue our reflective practice journey with a tool for personal practice before moving into learning about relational reflection.

ENGAGING IN PERSONAL REFLECTION

In 1999, Tema Okun published an article titled "White supremacy culture," identifying behaviors of white supremacy culture and their antidotes. Okun's article was part of her work on leading racial equity with training organizations and has expanded into her website, www.whitesupremacyculture.info, which I encourage you to check out. I will use some of these characteristics to deepen our individual reflective practice. The features of white supremacy highlighted below are fear, one right way, denial/defensiveness, and individualism. The characteristics of white supremacy are embedded into everything. They are the water we swim in and the air we breathe. Being an anti-oppressive practitioner is a lifetime journey. No easy path or finish line exists. As you read the section below, please journal, draw, or reflect on what you notice in your body and mind as you answer each question. In this section, I aim for you to ground deeply into your voice as a clinician who seeks to practice from an anti-oppressive framework. You may find that other questions arise for you. Take time to honor what you notice within yourself as we hold the thought that there is no one path or one way to justice and liberation.

Fear. Fear is that little voice in your head that says, *"You are messing up,"* or *"You will get into trouble if you do or ask X, Y, or Z."*

- How does fear show up for you as a provider to caregivers, young children, and babies? What do you notice in your body?

  _____

  _____

  _____

- What keeps you up at night?

  _____

  _____

  _____

- How do you imagine your fears impact the clinical relationship?

  _____

  _____

  _____

- How do they affect how you show up with clients and what you may choose to pay attention to as a client is sharing?

  _____

  _____

  _____

Some general topics that might bring fear up for providers are suicidality and scary thoughts that perinatal caregivers might share, such as intrusive thoughts about harm to the baby. As providers, we are responsible for supporting the well-being of the people we serve, and we also have punitive laws, like being mandated reporters. Calling CPS, involuntarily hospitalizing a client, or contacting the police for a welfare check are decisions that therapists have to make at one time or another. When high-intensity issues arise in counseling, clinicians must decide what actions to take. Reflective practice can help us recognize fear and face it. When a client shares something like *"I can't stop thinking about bringing a knife down to my belly,"* is my knee-jerk reaction to explore the possibility of hospitalization? If it is, can I recognize that this is my initial reaction and not necessarily the attuned response the client needs to hear? Initial reactions are part of the human experience. However, we have power over our next steps, like taking a breath, slowing down, and partnering with the client to understand more.

- When you notice discomfort, ask yourself: What is this feeling?
  This question is at the essence of reflective practice. Identifying our emotional experience is the first step to bringing awareness to the moment. Discomfort can be an emotional and also a physical feeling in our bodies. For many of us, discomfort might come with sensations in our chest, belly, or head. Where do you feel discomfort in your body? Attunement to your body can serve as a cue when a need to calm arises.

_____
_____
_____

- Where is the discomfort coming from?
  This question is about differentiating whether the discomfort or distress comes from our empathy for what the client is feeling or our fear. We can feel different things for different reasons. However, as we are the co-regulator in the client–provider relationship, figuring out what is happening inside us is vital.

  _____
  _____
  _____

- What does the discomfort mean? What is it trying to tell me?
  Discomfort is a cue that there is something needing attention. We might be tempted to push it away or dissociate from it, but insight comes from engaging in an internal dialogue. In a moment of high stress with a client, we may only have time to take one breath and say to ourselves, "*I see you. This is a lot.*" Sometimes, a brief acknowledgment is all we need. Attention to our internal world is the pathway towards attuning to others.

  _____
  _____
  _____

- How do I face the fear and be present for the client?
  This question moves us into action. While this may be a goal, action tends to be more productive when it is attuned to what we need at the moment. Without creating a brief moment to sit with our minds and bodies, we might risk jumping to a faulty solution. If we do, we can come back to these questions as a tool for reassessing the situation.

  _____
  _____
  _____

Fear can push us to look out for our well-being without considering the other(s). Its push is often outside awareness. In counseling, fear can be the voice that says we, as the provider, know what is best for the family. It can lead us to disconnect from families when we do not understand their cultural, relational, or spiritual practices. Sitting with fear is a skill developed over a lifetime. We will continuously experience many emotions as we provide services to clients. Our feelings give us information about what might be happening for the client. If my fear tells me that I might miss something and the client might harm their baby,

I can wonder how scared the client might be or about the fear and worry of their loved ones.

One right way. Okun explained that white supremacy holds the belief that "there is one right way to do things and once people are introduced to the right way, they will see the light and adopt it" (Okun, 1999, p. 4). Okun explains that the idea of one correct way of doing things aligns with values of perfectionism, paternalism, objectivity, and being qualified (Okun, n.d.). Notice the ways *one right way* shows up in your work and training. Have you ever been taught that there is one right way of doing therapy? Or of being ethical? The discourse of one way of practicing or that only specific interventions are helpful is alive in our field. Working with families brings the added complexity of caregiving practices. Reflection on our "correct behavior" ideas is vital to working with families.

- What feelings do you notice when you think about a family that parents or disciplines their children differently than yours?

  _____
  _____
  _____

- How are you partnering with families to determine what their right way is?

  _____
  _____
  _____

- What happens when you are unsure of what to do in a situation? Or when you do not have the answer?

  _____
  _____
  _____

- How loud is your inner critic?

  _____
  _____
  _____

- How do you define and judge your own mistakes?

  _____
  _____
  _____

Many immigrant Latine communities hold the value of respecting parents and elders. In the U.S. dominant culture, values of independence and autonomy move families to create more flexible space for children's feelings, as in the case of gentle parenting. We might come across a family that wants to balance validating their children's feelings while instilling cultural values of respect. We want to create space to understand the family's story. The space entails dialogue, observations, reflections, and more dialogue. Keeping the conversation open, checking hypotheses, and encouraging clients to evaluate what works for them are ways to partner and soothe our inner critic. The inner critic tries to tell us that we do not know what we are doing or any version of that statement. The reality is that we do not know until we partner with the other.

A therapist's relationship with a caregiver parallels the caregiver's relationship with their child.

- As a provider, how are you thinking about the power dynamics of parents and their children?

  _____
  _____
  _____

- How do you feel about the power dynamic between you and the caregiver?

  _____
  _____
  _____

- What questions are you asking yourself to recognize when paternalism appears in counseling?

  _____
  _____
  _____

- How are you creating space to reflect on your subjectivity to invite it into the clinical space?

  _____
  _____
  _____

Identities and power dynamics influence how we see the world and react to each other. Examining the dynamics present in our space is at the heart of anti-oppressive practice. It moves our work into an area that can promote equity and belonging. A racist discourse teaches that naming our differences leads to division. Naming is a step towards seeing and hearing the other. If I cannot name privileges, barriers, and history within myself, it becomes much harder to see it within the client.

These questions examine the myth of merit and the weight we give to a set of letters after someone's name. Education was my saving grace. It is how I breathed as I climbed out of the hole of darkness and despair. My education is valuable and signals my privilege. When I forget that my education does not mean complete insight into everything and everyone I support, I risk perpetuating harm.

- What does it mean to be qualified?

  _____
  _____
  _____

- Who gets to determine who is qualified?

  _____
  _____
  _____

- How are we honoring lived expertise in our understanding of professional experience?

  _____
  _____
  _____

- How are we creating space in our minds and the clinical relationship to explore what we do not know?

  _____
  _____
  _____

We all have blind spots. This truth is a reality of the human experience. The added layer of complexity is that, as therapists, we hold skills and tools that we share with families. We have some information to share, and so does the client. Providers must take a stance of curiosity in recognizing our ignorance as a remedy for thinking that there is only one way of navigating life. Ignorance is not a dirty word. It means that you and I still have more learning to do. When we recognize not knowing, we can move away from the idea that we will know and understand everything. We can partner, listen, and collaborate on solutions and how the clinical work will progress.

Denial and defensiveness. I invite you to imagine a situation where a client named a hurt or discomfort they felt about something you said or did. Notice what happens in your body when you think about being called in and called out.

- How does your social location impact the feelings and emotions that arise for you?

  _____
  _____
  _____

- How does it affect how others see and address you?

  _____
  _____
  _____

Notice what you imagine would arise for you as you sit with the client.

- What power dynamics (i.e., roles, intersectional identities) are at play?

  _____
  _____
  _____

- How was it for the client to experience the hurt or discomfort?

  _____
  _____
  _____

- How was it for them to share it with you?

  _____
  _____
  _____

- What do you need to do for yourself at this moment so that you can hear and hold what the client is sharing?

  _____
  _____
  _____

Denial and defensiveness can appear in many forms in our work with clients. It might be something the person is saying directly to us, or it may be something that triggers a wound in us. Let us dive into an example of this latter situation for clarity.

Mikaela is a perinatal clinician in her fifties working with Yamilet, a 25-year-old caregiver to twin babies. Yamilet explains that her mother abused her in childhood. She reports that she decided to stop communicating with her mother during pregnancy as she felt her mother was trying to "rule her life." Mikaela begins to ask Yamilet about her relationship with her mother and explores ways to restore the relationship.

Mikaela noticed that after the session, she was feeling frustrated at Yamilet. Reflecting on the session the next day, Mikaela began crying when she thought about Yamilet's mother. She thought, *"This generation does not care about family."* Mikaela has not spoken to her daughter in almost five years after her daughter left the family-of-origin home when she was 19. Mikaela can name for herself that the feelings of frustration and the ageist thoughts were related to the loss of her daughter. Mikaela now has an awareness of her emotions and their cause. She wonders whether her exploration of how Yamilet can restore the relationship with her mother was about meeting Yamilet's needs or about hers as the therapist. Mikaela makes a note to explore the misattunement of her recommendation with Yamilet in the next session. Imagine what might happen to Yamilet and Mikaela's relationship if the therapist did not have access to reflection.

Let us look at another example of defensiveness and denial. Yan is an East Asian caregiver in her thirties. She has been in counseling for three months with Darelys, a Caribbean Latina provider also in her thirties. Darelys spent today's session exploring the benefits of movement and spending time in nature as a tool for postpartum depression. Yan explained that she had been scared to go out, especially with the baby. Darelys asks Yan to share more about her fear. Yan explained that she had been scared to go out since witnessing a hate crime committed against an Asian person in 2021. Yan says, *"It's happened to so many people I know, and I just want to keep myself and my baby safe."* Darelys listened and encouraged Yan to engage in cognitive restructuring as a tool to manage fearful thoughts. Yan feels confused, angry, and misunderstood. However, she listens and follows the therapist's lead. When the telehealth session ends, Yan begins crying alone in her home.

- What did you notice in your body as you read this brief vignette?

  _____

  _____

  _____

- How did you notice that denial showed up in this example?

  _____

  _____

  _____

- What could have gone differently?

  _____

  _____

  _____

Denial can arise when we do not share the lived experience of the person we are supporting and have yet to work to educate ourselves on historical and present-day oppression. Knowing our social location is a remedy to accompany our reflection. Understanding our social location must involve vigilance of what we know and awareness that there will always be things we do not know. Having or knowing every experience is impossible (See Chapter 6 on cultural humility). The goal is not to be a perfect practitioner, as there is no such thing. The aim is to recognize that we will make mistakes, and when we make them, we are responsible for leaning into reflection and changing our behavior.

Individualism. Individualism holds the belief that we must do everything on our own. It can keep us in the space of thinking that we are constantly failing if we need support. The discourse of individualism can also give clinicians tunnel vision. We might find ourselves as providers wanting to push clients to thrive, strive, and become self-reliant. I invite you to notice what happens in your mind and body as you imagine an intergenerational home. In this home, you will find two grandmothers, two fathers, and their children: a 6-month-old baby and a 16-year-old daughter.

- What thoughts and feelings do you have about the role of a 16-year-old as related to the running of the household?

  _____
  _____
  _____

Imagine that the daughter is active in caring for the baby and responsible for picking up the baby from childcare.

- Has anything shifted inside of you as you think about this family?

  _____
  _____
  _____

- What if we add that this family is Afro-Latine?

  _____
  _____
  _____

- What shifts do you notice in your body?

  _____
  _____
  _____

- How does the clinical dynamic shift?

  _____
  _____
  _____

- What more must you know when considering the family's social positioning and culture?

  _____
  _____
  _____

Individualism can lead us to think that we do not need anyone else. It can lead a provider to stop consulting with a supervisor after obtaining licensure as if we become all-knowledgeable and fully aware of all countertransference once we meet that initial set of requirements. Consultation can help us see outside our worldview. A supervisor can support us in recognizing when we are re-enacting a situation with a client when we are triggered and do not even know it, and when we might be missing something. Collaboration can help us shine the light in the places we cannot see. It can move us away from the idea that we are supposed to know all the answers or figure things out alone. We were never meant to do any of this life stuff alone.

We learn, grow, and heal in the context of community. Sometimes individualism shows up in counseling with the "savior complex." White supremacy is the water we are all drinking, so it is easy to miss it when it shows up. I often hear clinicians sharing guilt and frustration at being unable to do more for clients. Some of the people we work with experience unimaginable pain. However, when we get stuck in a narrative of *"I must empower this person,"* we might lose sight of the person's inner strengths. People have been surviving long before we became their therapists. We must maintain sight and avoid getting stuck in the idea that we are the only ones who can help. Holding a balanced view of my role is a complex task for me. I care deeply about the people I work with and want to be useful, helpful, and a good therapist. Nevertheless, collaboration is the sweet spot of healing.

- How do you notice individualism in your work and identity as a mental health provider?

  _____
  _____
  _____

- How did your training as a provider and your specialties reinforce this value?

  _____
  _____
  _____

- What changes have you made to lean into collaboration?

  _____
  _____
  _____

You can bring reflection into your work as a clinician in these ways. I encourage you to consider the questions above and any others that come up for you as you work with clients. Please do not wait until a moment of discomfort arises. Remain vigilant about everything you notice as our experience filters our worldview. Everything you feel and experience in a relationship with a client might be a clue to your and the client's inner world. Our self-reflection will always have limits, as it relies on what we can see. Reflecting with other providers with a strong equity lens can give us space to see and hear what might be outside our awareness.

REFLECTIVE SUPERVISION/CONSULTATION

A reflective relationship is one of the most powerful tools for increasing aware-ness of our inner world. In trusting relationships, we can see parts of ourselves that are not always visible to us. I mentioned earlier that supervision should be integral to all clinicians' work lives. Many providers are familiar with clinical and administrative supervision from working in community mental health organiza-tions or meeting licensure requirements. Sometimes, our work with a supervisor might be connective and healing, while at other times it might feel like another check mark in the ocean of disconnected experiences. Reflective supervision/consultation (RS/C) is a professional relationship in the early relational health field that explores the provider's feelings and thoughts as they support families with babies and young children (Alliance for the Advancement of Infant Mental Health, 2018). In introducing RS/C in this text, I hope that providers can connect with a supervisor or consultant to support the *heart parts* of this work.

One of the greatest gifts of RS/C is its focus on the parallel process. Heffron and Murch (2010) defined the parallel process as "the interlocking network of relationships between supervisor, supervisees, families, and children" (p. 9). RS/C is a tool that can help providers examine, understand, and impact how caregivers interact with themselves and with their little ones. Through the lens of the parallel process, a supervisor's relationship with their supervisee impacts how that super-visee holds and interacts with the caregiver. In turn, the supervisee's relationship with the caregiver affects how that caregiver interacts with their children. Another marker of RS/C is an emphasis on attuning to our inner wisdom. Instead of clini-cal supervision, where we might discuss specific strategies with clinicians, RS/C moves us to sit with self-awareness and internal knowledge, honoring Tenets on self-awareness and the importance of non-dominant knowledge (Alliance for the Advancement of Infant Mental Health, 2018; Tenets Initiative, 2018). This supervi-sion model entails reflection, collaboration, and regularity. Each component con-tributes to the other and contributes to developing trust and depth.

Reflection

Reflection entails supporting the provider to bring awareness to their internal experience. The supervisor guides the clinician to recognize and question the feelings and thoughts that emerge as they sit with families. Supervisees strengthen their reflective capacity by slowing down and examining their internal responses. Inner exploration helps providers explore the potential experience for each family member. Let us look at an example.

Nira is a clinician in her early forties working with Marcus, a 36-year-old father to 1-year-old Anaya. Marcus sought counseling due to experiencing symptoms of postnatal depression. Nira and Marcus have worked together weekly for the past three months. Nira is receiving RS/C from Yerutí, and they have been working together for two years. During today's RS/C, Nira shared that Marcus disclosed feeling disconnected from Anaya during this week's session. Yerutí noticed that Nira seemed to be staring at the floor as she shared about the session and that her affect seemed flat, which was uncharacteristic. Yerutí asked Nira about what it was like for her to be with the family during this session. Nira became tearful and shared concern about Anaya growing up without a father. Upon further exploring Nira's experience, she shared sadness regarding her postpartum period. Nira shared that depression kept her feeling disconnected from her last child until she was 9 months old. She connected her experience with postpartum depression with her reaction to Marcus. This insight helped Nira gain a deeper understanding of Marcus and Anaya's experiences. RS/C helps practitioners understand how each relationship impacts the other and intentionally connect our lived experience with the lived expertise of others (Alliance for the Advancement of Infant Mental Health, 2018). We welcome all of who we are, knowing that our experience filters what we do and how we are.

Collaboration

Collaboration is an aspect of RS/C that expands our capacity to deepen reflection. The supervisor and supervisee aim to develop a mutually satisfying dynamic by working together. The parties involved think together and respect work and commitment to supporting families (Heffron & Murch, 2010). The collaboration moves the relationship away from other directive and expert-focused models. The supervisor facilitates this process by encouraging the co-creation of the space, goals, and exploration. Attunement is a tool to foster collaboration. The supervisor takes steps to slow down, understand, and ensure they follow the supervisee's lead. The constant synchronization to the supervisee's needs and experience creates a holding environment. The relationship between the reflective collaborators becomes a place that mirrors the therapist's work with the family. To illustrate, let us continue with Nira's example.

Nira and Yerutí are now about halfway into their supervision time. Yerutí noticed that she did not ask Nira what she hoped to discuss in this meeting to co-create the agenda. Yerutí waits for a space in the meeting to ensure that she attunes to Nira's needs. She says, *"I realize that we are halfway into our meeting, and I didn't check in with you about what you wanted to discuss today before starting. How is this conversation feeling for you? Is there anything else you would like for us to make time for?"* Nira reflects on how she did not realize the feelings that stirred up for her during the session with Marcus. She asks Yerutí, *"What should I do next time?"* In honoring the principle of collaboration, Yerutí invites Nira to think together about her next steps with the family.

Regularity

Predictability can help us build a sense of trust. The regularity of RS/C helps create an environment where the supervisor can meet the supervisee's needs, creating "an opportunity for ongoing discussion on all aspects of the work" (Heffron & Murch, 2010, p. 7). Regularity also gives the relationship and the parties involved a sense that they are valuable to each other. Each reflective collaborator has a dedicated and protected time for each other. Parallel to the counseling experience, we want shifts in the schedule of RS/C to be minimal. Imagine how different the dynamic between Yerutí and Nira would be if they only met on an as-needed basis. Would there be enough trust for Nira to have shared her experience? Would Yerutí have noticed that Nira was feeling some kind of way (i.e., displeased, uncomfortable, etc.) about the session with Marcus?

RS/C is a seemingly simple yet complex framework for supporting providers. It is a relational learning model where providers experience "being with" and "being held." It requires a move away from the push to develop solutions and jump into action. Instead, this model asks practitioners to slow down, notice what arises, and consider the meaning, relationships, and storylines as tools for developing insight and exploring hypotheses with families. Although RS/C helps to increase reflective capacity, it has not been established as a space to examine implicit biases and social justice (Lingras, 2021). The following section presents some shifts in the RS/C field that support AOT.

RS/C AS A TOOL FOR ADVANCING SOCIAL JUSTICE

In his book *Race talk and the conspiracy of silence*, Deral Wing Sue (2015) outlined why our society avoids interracial race-based dialogues. Sue explained that race-related topics tend to bring intense emotions into the room. Discourses on keeping the status quo and being polite mar our society. When people introduce uncomfortable conversations, they break the unspoken societal rules around politeness and avoiding discomfort. As discomfort arises in groups, individuals might want to switch topics or "agree to disagree." This strategy is a way of maintaining the politeness protocol and the dominant narrative. It sends the message that discomfort is bad and needs to go away. Okun (1999) also discussed a perceived right to comfort and avoidance of conflict as characteristics of white supremacy culture. Clinicians looking to implement an AOT stance into RS/C must invite race and other identities into the room. Race and racism are always present, and our avoidance of the topic colludes with racism.

Supervisors and supervisees can practice creating a space that welcomes discussions on social location, implicit biases, intersectionality, and critical reflection (Indigo Cultural Center, 2022). When we consistently and mindfully invite these conversations into RS/C, we can collectively change the discourse of unconditional validation. Whether we like it or not, when we avoid addressing harmful material during discussions, we create space to welcome it. This action might leave the unintentional message that it is acceptable to hold oppressive beliefs. Sometimes, in the search for *meeting people where they are* or attuning to the supervisee's needs, we may fail to expand on a conversation or question something that profoundly relates to structural inequalities. The Tenets (2018) invite us to engage in difficult conversations around race and other forms of oppression. They encourage us to hold self-awareness, consider our stance on diversity-informed care, understand the macro-level impact, and advance equitable policy. We can use them as a guide to relational learning. Reflective collaborators can have them present during RS/C. They can ask questions like, *"Which Tenet are we noticing in this conversation?" "What Tenet did we leave out as we explore the identities present between you and the family? Between us [supervisor–supervisee]?"*

There are many ways to hold AOT during our work. The main factor is that we must be intentional. Whether we address it or not, race and power dynamics are always present in every space. Those who hold dominant identities must remain vigilant of our relationship with comfort, race talk, and oppression.

SUMMARY

Healing begins when we show up as our most authentic selves in a space that welcomes our fullness. Through reflective practice, we can create that space within us and in relationships with supervisors and consultants. A model for relational reflection that stems from early relational health practice is RS/C. RS/C with an AOT lens calls us to notice how white supremacy culture and other dominant lenses inform our work, thoughts, and feelings. The more we can lean into discomfort, the more we expand towards growth. Our best tool for reflection is curiosity about our inner world and what happens in the space between us and others. We can use the Tenets as a guide to explore our awareness and attunement to the diversity within RS/C.

REFERENCES

Alliance for the Advancement of Infant Mental Health. (2018). Best practice guidelines for reflective supervision/consultation. https://tinyurl.com/3k8faf3c

Bhola, P., Duggal, C., & Isaac, R. (2022). *Reflective practice and professional development in psychotherapy*. Sage.

DeAngelis, T. (2019). Better relationships with patients lead to better outcomes. *Monitor on Psychology*, (*50*)10. https://www.apa.org/monitor/2019/11/ce-corner-relationships

Erikson Institute. (2015, May). FAN tool developed by Erikson's Fussy Baby Network becomes a national model. https://tinyurl.com/mzvsjykt

Gilkerson, L., & Imberger, J. (2016). *Strengthening reflective capacity in skilled home visitors*. Zero to Three.

Heffron, M. C., & Murch, T. (2010). *Reflective supervision and leadership in infant and early childhood programs*. Zero to Three.

Heller, S. S., & Gilkerson, L. (2009). *A practical guide to reflective supervision*. Zero to Three.

Hook, J. N., Farrell, J. E., Davis, D. E., DeBlaere, C., Van Tongeren, D. R., & Utsey, S. O. (2016). Cultural humility and racial microaggressions in counseling. *Journal of Counseling Psychology*, *63*(3), 269–277. https://doi.org/10.1037/cou0000114

Indigo Cultural Center. (2022). Digging deeper: De-colonizing our understanding and practice of reflective supervision through a racial equity lens. https://tinyurl.com/2bpmdryw

Lingras, K. A. (2021). Mind the gap(s): Reflective supervision/consultation as a mechanism for addressing implicit bias and reducing our knowledge gaps. *Infant Mental Health Journal*, *43*(4), 638–652. https://doi.org/10.1002/imhj.21993

Okun, T. (1999). White supremacy culture. https://www.whitesupremacyculture.info/uploads/4/3/5/7/43579015/okun_-_white_sup_culture_2020.pdf

Okun, T. (n.d.). White supremacy characteristics. https://www.whitesupremacy culture.info/characteristics.html

Pawl, J. H., & St. John, M. (1998). *How you are is as important as what you do … in making a positive difference for infants, toddlers, and their families*. Zero to Three.

Priddis, L., & Rogers, S. L. (2017). Development of the reflective practice questionnaire: Preliminary findings. *Reflective Practice*, *19*(1), 89–104. https://doi.org/10.1080/14623943.2017.1379384

Sakamoto, I., & Pitner, R. O. (2005). Use of critical consciousness in anti-oppressive social work practice: Disentangling power dynamics at personal and structural levels. *British Journal of Social Work*, *35*(4), 435–452. https://doi.org/10.1093/bjsw/bch190

Strier, R., & Biyamin, S. (2014). Introducing anti-oppressive social work practices in public services: Rhetoric to practice. *British Journal of Social Work* 44(8), 2095–2112. https://doi.org/10.1093/bjsw/bct049

Sue, D. W. (2015). *Race talk and the conspiracy of silence*. Wiley.

Tenets Initiative. (2018). Diversity-informed tenets for work with infants, children & families/Principios informados en la diversidad para trabajar con bebés, niños, niñas y familias. Irving Harris Foundation. https://diversityinformedtenets.org/download-the-tenets/

CHAPTER SIX

Aspiring to Embody Cultural Humility

Tervalon and Murray-Garcia developed the term and practice of cultural humility in 1998. Their work called the healthcare fields to move into curiosity and humbleness about experiences outside of ourselves. They noticed that teachings on cultural competency focused on memorizing different stereotypical behavioral expectations from individuals of minoritized racial and ethnic groups. Many training programs continue to teach healthcare providers a set of often harmful expectations from non-dominant communities (Sini, 2017). For example, most of my training in providing culturally appropriate services entailed cultural competency. Many of my textbooks and coursework referenced stereotypical and often harmful beliefs about other cultures, such as framing familial relationships among Latino people as enmeshed. Cultural competence aims to support providers in working with diverse populations. However, it misses the embodiment of humility, which is critical to reflection and changing our views (Pallato, 2019; Sloane et al., 2018). The more I reflected and learned about myself in community with others, the more interested I became in becoming anti-racist and anti-oppressive. My journey entailed digging into anti-racist content (books and videos) and deepened in working with an anti-racist coach. In 2022, I completed my doctorate in social work focused on cultural humility in the perinatal period. This chapter shares some of my research findings, reflections, and techniques for embodying cultural humility in clinical practice.

CULTURAL HUMILITY

Cultural humility entails a lifelong commitment to self-reflection and critique of our beliefs, implicit biases, power dynamics, and communication (Tervalon &

DOI: 10.4324/9781003286394-8

Murray-Garcia, 1998). Our capacity to hold humility and curiosity when working with perinatal caregivers and their children is vital to building connection and reducing the likelihood of causing harm. Humility is a way of being that recognizes the limits of our knowledge and experience. It serves as a reminder that the expert's role is narrow and often wrong. Our mental health training, while valuable, comes from a dominant and Eurocentric lens. Leaning into a humble spirit can help us build a capacity to tolerate the unknown and the reality of making mistakes. Humility is the bridge to curiosity, which allows us to question our assumptions. We all make assumptions about others and the world. However, individuals and families are complex. Experiences with our family of origin, friends, peers, community, and political system, among others, inform our worldview. Our worldview constantly impacts our understanding of everything we perceive. As outlined in Tenet 1, self-awareness is vital to embodying cultural humility (Tenets Initiative, 2018). Think about the messages you received in your upbringing about what it meant to be a good person, parent, and provider.

- How are those messages present in your daily life?

  _____
  _____
  _____

- How have you adjusted or leaned into early messages to advance social justice in your practice?

  _____
  _____
  _____

As we explore cultural humility, you will find some commonalities between this chapter and Chapter 5 on reflective practice. The main common ground is that being anti-oppressive requires intentional reflection. It starts inward with the "I."

Therapists bring their whole-selves into the clinical relationship and ways of supporting clients. What we think, feel, and hold on to impacts how we show up and our capacity to create space for others. Critical self-awareness and critique of our values, beliefs, and experiences can help us remain conscious of the limits of our understanding (Sloane et al., 2018). We cannot be aware of every blind spot, but when we are open to the possibility of their existence in our minds, we can wonder about their presence in decision-making.

- What and whose view does my thinking represent?
- What view is missing?
- What steps must I take to look outside of my limited individual perspective?

Constantly wondering what we may not see is a cornerstone of cultural humility. It also means that we honor the reality of not knowing. In this way of being, we embody the classic statement: *We don't know what we don't know until we know it*. Part of our work as clinicians is supporting people to become aware of the different aspects of themselves impacting decision-making. Using an object-relations framework, we help clients gain insight into their internal relationships (Frankland, 2010). When we bring cultural humility, we turn our eyes inward and look at what might be missing from our understanding as providers.

Cultural humility is also a way of being stemming from transformation inside and outside the counseling space. Therapists hold a reflective stance as we sit with clients. We wonder how our experience influences our perception of what we think we understand. Bringing this transformation outside the counseling space means that we live cultural humility. Aspiring to embodying cultural humility entails maintaining curiosity and an anti-oppressive stance in all parts of our lives. It requires us to think about cultural humility in everything we do. One of my favorite explanations of the concept is in an article by Foronda et al. (2016, p. 214), which states:

> [C]ultural humility implies one must strive for learning at the highest level of learning; that of transformation [Mezirow, 2003]. Cultural humility involves a change in overall perspective and way of life … This process will not happen immediately, but it is speculated that with time, education, reflection, and effort, progress can be made.

Transformational learning is an adult learning theory that focuses on changing problematic ways of thinking (Mezirow, 2003). Through transformation, individuals shift rigid beliefs and habitual patterns of thought. Embarking on the cultural humility journey entails constantly challenging our ways of thinking and behaving. We might challenge discourses about patient care and what it means to be a good human. For example, providers may wonder how we understand the commonly used terms *compliance* and *resistance*. Who determines if a client is compliant, and what that means? How are we considering intersectional dynamics in our understanding of compliance? What interactions do we imagine when thinking about a compliant client or family? How are dominant views impacting this definition? How does the client understand our meaning and expectation of compliance?

Let us reflect on anti-oppression outside the counseling room.

- How are anti-oppressive ways of being showing up in other areas of our lives?

  _____

  _____

  _____

- When we look at our social circles, who do we see represented?

  _____

  _____

  _____

- What content do we consume? Sit back and notice what is missing.
  o   How are you making sense of it?

  _____

  _____

  _____

- Who and what do we support? Is it aligned with who you are in a work setting?

  _____

  _____

  _____

Applying cultural humility will look different for everyone because there is no one way to be anti-oppressive. However, reflection and action are always in the mix.

- What are you doing to be culturally humble in your everyday life?

We recognize that racism, homophobia, transphobia, ableism, and other forms of oppression are not something that is *over there* impacting other people. We might read a book, listen to a talk, attend a training, and think, *"This would be great for my team/boss/neighbor to hear."* We disconnect from the work as if it does not apply to us. However, racism and oppression are right *here*, within me and you. The sooner we can see this reality, the sooner we can embark on our aspiration to be anti-racist and culturally humble.

A REFLECTION ON MY WHY

I decided to complete a doctorate in social work for many different reasons. The first reason is that it was a life goal. A part of me is constantly aiming to be and feel good enough. In the years before leaving Venezuela, there was a narrative my mom told me. It became a sort of mantra: *"Vas a estudiar en los Estados Unidos"* (You are going to study in the United States), *"Voy a estudiar en los Estados Unidos"* (I am going to study in the United States). I remember the night before leaving my home in Venezuela so clearly. I was 10 years old. It was evening time, and I was looking out the window of my room in a third-floor apartment.

I could see the mountains far off to my right. That evening, alone at my window, I talked to the country, my friends, the mountains, the sky, and the moon. I let them know that I would be leaving and would not be returning. I told them I would miss them but that it would be okay because I would study in the United States. It is a moment cemented in my mind. If I close my eyes, I can smell the air of that evening. I felt a sense of loneliness and deep knowing that everything would change. I tried to hold on to hope. Hope is something we do as humans. For me, resilience came from a deep place of holding on to the hope that my life could be better. In my most painful moments, I knew *this* could not be it. I refused to believe that this was what my life would look like. To be clear, there was pain even amid hope, and the combination of hope, opportunity, and privilege helped me survive.

Sometimes, the pain swallowed the hope, but it always came back. I share this because this is part of my reflection on my journey. It is part of my *why*. Education was the hope I hung on to. I am still determining whether embarking on a doctorate program is the culmination of this wish to study in the United States, a desire for others to see me as competent, or knowing what is possible and where I can make a change. It could be part of trying to feel like I belong in a world not created for me. Most likely, it is a combination of everything.

One of the other reasons for embarking on this journey was a desire to find the common denominator in what causes suffering. My goal in life is to support a world where we do not have to spend our adulthood healing from the wounds of childhood. Psychosocial stressors like untreated parental mental health conditions create risk. Yet, what I know to be true is that most perinatal caregivers experiencing mental health complications do not abuse their children. On the contrary, I see caregivers who feel at their worst and still show up for their children. I am in awe of the families I met along the way. As someone with 10+ ACES (accounting for Urban ACES), partnering with families and witnessing love is soul healing. It also left me with the question of finding common ground. If it was not an untreated mental health condition, what the heck was it?

I am not exactly sure how it happened, but once I saw the reality of racism and oppression, I could not unsee it. I saw how this system that is always at play had impacted my life, and I had not seen it. I thought it was me, that I was bad. I believed that something was so profoundly wrong with me that all injustices in my life made sense. There is a theory for the awareness or awakening I experienced: Liberation psychology. This theory refers to developing a critical consciousness of the oppression we experience (Comas-Díaz & Torres Rivera, 2020). Colonization stole my ancestors' capacity to build an internal sense of safety and roots in our family and land. I was not accepted in Venezuela as a Venezuelan because my family members were immigrants there. I do not meet the ideal picture some people have when they think of a Venezuelan.

Xenophobia was always a part of my life. I am grateful to be in the U.S.A., and I can also say that life here is hard for immigrants. I see a bi-directional relationship between interpersonal trauma and systemic oppression. I wonder how much different my childhood would have been if my family had access to internal and external resources. Would I have been abused? Would I have felt as lonely? Would my caregiver's experience of me and my sibling be different? What about my caregiver's capacity to be present for us? Would life have been different for her? I am not sure. As survivors, we can be good at sitting in *what-if* scenarios. We can collectively say that racism, colonization, and oppression create impossible situations for families and caregivers. They chisel away hope, patience, and understanding. They create danger, sorrow, and constant heartache. They are the systems that poison the well we all drink from.

I share this reflection because we can only do this work with a deep understanding of our history and who we are. The more we reflect, the more we see and learn. We discover patterns that require nurturing and others that need change. Applying a critical lens is the work of cultural humility. It is constant, unrelenting, and filled with heart. Before I share about my research, I want to share this quote from Ruth King (2016, para. 13) to help us get grounded in our *why*:

> We must be clear in our intentions regarding what we want to wake up to, and then attend to them mindfully. We all need an intention beyond righteousness. Ask yourself, what is your vision of racial healing? Why is this important to you personally? What do you need to face up to and own in order to stay awake to racial suffering? How would this benefit all beings?

I encourage you to spend some time here sitting in reflection. You may journal, draw, or notice what comes up for you.

CULTURAL HUMILITY IN PERINATAL SOCIAL WORK

My doctoral study was qualitative action research on social workers' understanding of cultural humility (Velasquez, 2022). I wanted to understand how mental health providers conceptualized and applied the concept. My research question was, "How can perinatal social workers apply cultural humility?" As my doctorate program was in social work (DSW), I collected information from fellow social workers. My study was small, as it included 14 participants from three different groups: Perinatal social workers, providers who train perinatal social workers, and social work educators. A small study with a specific population brings challenges and opportunities. The challenge is that we need more research to understand these concepts across populations and disciplines.

A strength is that it allows for a specialized focus on serving perinatal clients. We can talk about cultural humility, but its application in work with clients can remain abstract for many.

I found four major themes in my research from my interviews with the participants: (1) Deciding to move beyond cultural competency, (2) applying an anti-oppressive lens, (3) integrating foundational social work skills, and (4) addressing training challenges. The themes represent possible pathways for being culturally humble with perinatal clients. Other viewpoints fall outside my study's boundaries and may be subjects for future research. My investigation centers specifically on the four themes listed above. Practitioners can apply a critical lens to the themes and results to support their work with perinatal families. You can review the executive summary in the Appendix for more information. I encourage providers to continue their journey by expanding their learning with other sources.

Deciding to Move Beyond Cultural Competency

The balance between competence and humility entails shifting who we see as experts. Through a lens of competence, therapists bring their knowledge base of the client's culture and values into conceptualizing the problem. A humility framework calls on us to center the client's lived expertise and to recognize them as the cultural expert. Therapists must find ways to integrate cultural humility into their training and supervision. I envision a time when cultural humility will be part of everything we do. However, this is not our reality, meaning that providers must do the work to examine what they are learning. Here's a simple example. We have all been to a training on trauma or trauma-informed care. How many of those trainings named the importance of considering historical trauma? Another critical piece to moving beyond competence is engaging in constant self-reflection. This book offers multiple reflective questions you can use before and after interactions with clients and other providers. When we honor "Self-awareness leads to better services" we can examine our stance towards families, how resources are allocated, and what we do regarding advocacy (Tenets Initiative, 2018, para. 1). Action without awareness risks harm.

Equitable change can only happen when the players in power are taking the steps necessary to challenge their ways of thinking and being. We are the players in power in the client–therapist relationship, as it contains an internal hierarchy. Providers often serve as gatekeepers in the field. For instance, how can we recognize and respect non-dominant bodies of knowledge (Tenet 4) without examining our reaction when non-dominant ways of thinking appear? The recognition of our inner world moves performative action into an embodiment. I often get asked in trainings: How do I avoid performative allyship? I think the answer is we must live and breathe authenticity. The motivation behind performative allyship is to accrue status and resources to satisfy our needs rather than a true focus on the group we seek to support (Kutlaca & Radke, 2022). It is a sneaky concept. One can work to create changes that seem helpful from the outside but maintain the status quo of those in privileged positions.

An example might be someone who advocates for affordable housing but opposes the program in their neighborhood because of concern that their property value will decrease. The advocacy for affordable housing represents an attempt towards allyship, while the performative aspect is not wanting to lose power. Is who I am on the outside the same as on the inside? For me, that is imperfect, messy, silly, and passionate, among other characteristics. Being a "good" person is an idea that is deeply embedded in our society, so none of us are immune from *performativeness*. Authenticity requires intentionality. How is your inside cultural humility journey matching your outside one?

Applying an Anti-Oppressive Lens

Cultural humility is an anti-oppressive framework. My research identified several steps providers could take to sharpen their anti-oppressive lens: Increasing awareness of structural racism and systemic oppression, awareness of biases, the impact of social location, awareness of ethnocentrism, and applying an intersectional lens. Let us briefly look at each of them below.

Increasing awareness of structural racism and systemic oppression. Our history helps us understand the present. We cannot look at current social problems like poverty and access to care without understanding how colonization, structural racism, and other forms of oppression impact people. Part of the reason I recall history in each aspect of this text is that it helps bring awareness of the powers at play. We can better support an immigrant Brown family whose child is experiencing behavioral concerns when we can see (1) how Brown children and their parents are treated in the school systems, (2) how immigrant communities are treated in the school system, and (3) how bureaucracy creates barriers to work, like what kinds of jobs are accessible for undocumented individuals, among many other questions. There is also a remedy for providers to take action in learning about systemic racism and other forms of oppression. This action calls us to consume content outside traditional mental health material, which does not always reference history. The remedy reflects the Tenet "Recognize and respect non-dominant bodies of knowledge" (Tenets Initiative, 2018, para. 4).

Awareness of biases. Awareness of systemic racism can be a starting point for examining our biases. The stance towards infants, children, and families for the diversity-informed practice section of the Tenets (2018) has four areas that can help bring light to our biases. Tenet 2 calls us to "Champion Children's Rights Globally." If we see children as citizens of the world, what are we doing to support and nurture them? How are we holding children in mind in our decision-making? I am talking beyond the children we might be raising. I am inviting you to think about your values. How are we supporting perinatal caregivers? Are we unintentionally or intentionally creating barriers to caregivers' access to services?

Providers are responsible for examining our practices and policies and their impact on the people we serve (Tenets Initiative, 2018). How are we using our privilege to combat discrimination (Tenet 3)? At the beginning of my career, I navigated the world by keeping my head down and my mouth shut. I was scared, and I did not want to be the troublemaker. As I step into leadership, I recognize that part of my bias is fear-driven and that this is an area I must constantly work on strengthening so that my inside can match my outside. When we notice harmful practices in our work or organization, what are we doing to change the practices or to call others into conversation?

Tenet 4 calls us to recognize that research and evidence-based practices only hold some answers to serve the complexities of the human experience (Tenets Initiative, 2018). We must reach outside them to obtain a more comprehensive picture.

- What do you notice inside your body when you think of a non-dominant way of practicing healing?

  _____

  _____

  _____

- When the client names what supports them and is different from our spiritual or any other value system, how are we to understand any discomfort that may arise for us?

  _____

  _____

  _____

- What is your reaction when you see a training based on a practice not deemed evidence-based?

  _____

  _____

  _____

Awareness of biases reminds us to lean into the Tenet "Honor diverse family structures" (Tenets Initiative, 2018, para. 5). Close your eyes and think of a family. This family has two preschool-aged children and two caregivers. One of the caregivers works as a stay-at-home parent, while the other works outside the home. What do you notice about what comes up regarding the makeup of this family? How are we partnering with the family to understand their structure?

Impact of social location. Our social location impacts our access to power. As I mentioned in previous chapters, we have a sacred responsibility to use our privilege for the benefit of others. How do you understand your proximity to whiteness? This question is vital for someone like me with advanced Vitiligo and others with lighter skin colors. Whether we like it or not, how others view us makes a difference. We have to see color, and we have to see other historically marginalized identities. Sue (2015) explained in his book *Race talk and the conspiracy of silence* that "as long as one professes color blindness, race talk is avoided and muted" (p.77). When we avoid conversations, we silence and further harm. This point is directly related to the characteristic of white supremacy, the need for comfort, mentioned in Chapter 5. Frequently, when we avoid being discomforted, we make others feel uncomfortable. Those of us with marginalized identities, especially Black and Indigenous communities, are usually constantly uncomfortable in dominant spaces. My awareness of social location can help me understand where I hold privilege and where I experience marginalization.

Awareness of ethnocentrism. Our practices, Codes of Ethics, and interventions are filtered through a Eurocentric lens. Ethnocentrism refers to our tendency to place our experience at the center of everything, evaluating others through our perspective (Oeberst & Matschke, 2017). The way we do things is familiar and comfortable for us. An ethnocentric view can be so ingrained in our value system that when faced with another way of doing it, we might jump into thinking it is wrong. The following is a scenario to illustrate.

Ayana, who is six months pregnant, visits a therapist, as she is concerned about increased anxiety. Ayana and the therapist are from two different racial and ethnic backgrounds. In this first session with the therapist, Ayana shares that she struggles to balance her family's expectations. Ayana worries about her extended family's involvement after her baby arrives. The therapist focused the session on collecting information and completing the biopsychosocial assessment. Towards the end of the session, the therapist comments, *"It's important to set boundaries with your family. Independence and well-being are interconnected."* Ayana seems confused, as she did not mention a need for independence. The therapist continues, *"We can work together to figure out ways to improve your communication and ensure your needs are met."* In this example, the provider's response reflects ethnocentrism. A remedy here is to get into the habit of asking: How is ethnocentrism present in this conversation or way of thinking? A second step is collaborating with clients and communities to ensure we co-create and shift strategies based on what people tell us they need and how to meet those needs.

Applying an intersectional lens. Kimberly Crenshaw (1989) coined the theory of intersectionality following her experiences supporting Black women in navigating the legal system. Intersectionality offers a framework to understand how different identities merge and impact the barriers we face as we navigate the world. Clinicians must examine the impact of the intersections of being a caregiver, an individual, and any other identities present for that person.

Integrating Foundational Practice Skills

I re-titled this section for this chapter from its original theme, "Integrating foundational social work skills." As a social worker, my foundational skills are centered on the client's self-determination, prioritizing cultural needs, and practicing at the micro-/mezzo-/macro-levels. I encourage you here to become familiarized with your field and its foundational skills.

- What can you bring from the foundational skills in your discipline into your practice of cultural humility?

_____

_____

_____

- What do you know about the history of your field and what it holds as essential?

_____

_____

_____

- How can you examine those skills and techniques through a critical lens so that you can build on what is already there?

_____

_____

_____

I learned the phrase _retrofit_ in a training on reproductive justice led by Monica McLemore in 2022. McLemore described the term as taking something already available and adapting it to meet our needs (i.e., health and birth equity). In our case, we might be retrofitting ways to advance social justice through infusing cultural humility into our existing practices.

Addressing Training Challenges

Training challenges involve multiple realms. The first aspect is ensuring we learn from individuals with lived experience. This step is vital to centering the needs of silenced communities. If I want to know about ableism, I need to do the work to learn from individuals impacted by ableism. I want to acknowledge that many of us may not be members of historically marginalized groups, yet we are deeply dedicated to serving the community. However, if we are going to truly own this shifting of power, we have to do some things differently. The most visible content and trainings are those led by individuals and organizations with higher access to power and privilege. We can collectively live the Tenet, "Make space and open pathways," by questioning learning opportunities that lack diversity, advocating for representation, supporting the work of people with lived experience, and recognizing when we might need to take a step back and listen (Tenets Initiative, 2018, para. 9).

Another challenge mentioned by participants is the gap between theory and practice. Clinicians need access to supervision to implement what we are learning. We learn by doing, which can lead to harm if not properly supported. Lack of appropriate support can harm the people we work with and us as providers. We risk burning out when we do not have the resources we need. Support and training must be accessible and come in different forms. We need organizations to honor non-dominant bodies of knowledge. I understand that advanced certifications and programs are critical to adequate care and that they create barriers. I constantly walk this line of wanting to offer content that is accessible and recognizing that my career is my livelihood. It is how I pay my bills and how I hope to be able to buy a home one day. At the same time, I wonder if we can collectively find a middle ground where we are honoring our needs and those of the communities we are part of and serve. I do not know what that can look like for you. However, my balance is to offer my heart-quality content at three tiers, from free to higher fee. Again, this is not perfect. Our world is not calling us to perfection. It calls us to think outside the box of what we have been taught is possible and acceptable.

For more information, please check out my doctoral program deliverable, *Cultural humility in perinatal social work: A toolkit for professionals*, in the Appendix.

SUMMARY

Applying cultural humility is complex. It requires knowing our field, history, and ourselves. It asks us to engage in an anti-oppressive way of being and navigating the world. When we lean into this journey, we find that there must be a congruence between our inner world and what we do. Without congruence, we risk moving into performative allyship that further harms ourselves and those we aim to support. Critical reflection is the bridge to cultural humility. My research is a resource that mental health providers can use to explore and continue to expand their learning on cultural humility in perinatal services. I encourage providers to take what works and leave what does not as they apply a critical lens to the study's four themes: (1) Deciding to move beyond cultural competency, (2) using an anti-oppressive lens, (3) integrating foundational social work skills, and (4) addressing training challenges.

REFERENCES

Comas-Díaz, L., & Torres Rivera, E. (2020). *Liberation psychology: Theory, method, practice, and social justice*. American Psychological Association.

Crenshaw, K. (1989). Demarginalizing the intersection of race and sex: A Black feminist critique of antidiscrimination doctrine, feminist theory and antiracist politics. *University of Chicago Legal Forum*, *1*(8). 139–167. https://chicagounbound.uchicago.edu/uclf/vol1989/iss1/8

Foronda, C., Baptiste, D. L., Reinholdt, M. M., & Ousman, K. (2016). Cultural humility: A concept analysis. *Journal of Transcultural Nursing: Official Journal of the Transcultural Nursing Society*, *27*(3), 210–217. https://doi.org/10.1177/1043659615592677

Frankland, A. G. (2010). *The little psychotherapy book: Object relations in practice*. Oxford University Press.

King, R. (2016, June 5). Being mindful of race. https://ruthking.net/being-mindful-of-race/

Kutlaca, M., & Radke, H. R. (2022). Toward an understanding of performative allyship: Definition, antecedents, and consequences. *Social and Personality Psychology Compass*, *17*(2), 1–12. https://doi.org/10.1111/spc3.12724

Mezirow, J. (2003). Transformative learning as discourse. *Journal of Transformative Education*, *1*(1). 58–63. https://doi.org/10.1177/1541344603252172

Oeberst, A., & Matschke, C. (2017). Word order and world order: Titles of intergroup conflicts may increase ethnocentrism by mentioning the in-group first. *Journal of Experimental Psychology: General*, *146*(5), 672–690. https://doi.org/10.1037/xge0000300.supp

Pallato, B. A. (2019). The multicultural guidelines in practice: Cultural humility in clinical training and supervision. *Training and Education in Professional Psychology*, *13*(3), 227–232. https://doi.org/10.1037/tep0000253

Sini, R. (2017, October 20). Publisher apologizes for "racist text" in medical book. https://www.bbc.com/news/blogs-trending-41692593

Sloane, H. M., David, K., Davies, J., Stamper, D., & Woodward, S. (2018). Cultural history analysis and professional humility: Historical context and social work practice. *Social Work Education*, *37*(8), 1015–1027. https://doi.org/10.1080/02615479.2018.1490710

Sue, D. W. (2015). *Race talk and the conspiracy of silence: Understanding and facilitating difficult dialogues on race*. Wiley.

Tenets Initiative. (2018). Diversity-informed tenets for work with infants, children & families/Principios informados en la diversidad para trabajar con bebés, niños, niñas y familias. Irving Harris Foundation. https://diversityinformedtenets.org/download-the-tenets/

Tervalon, M., & Murray-Garcia, J. (1998). Cultural humility versus cultural competence: A critical distinction in defining physician training outcomes in multicultural education. *Journal of Health Care for the Poor and Underserved*, *9*(2), 117–125. https://doi.org/10.1353/hpu.2010.0233

Velasquez, M. (2022). Cultural humility in perinatal social work: A toolkit for professionals. https://tinyurl.com/3ykvj2b7

Conducting Assessments

CHAPTER SEVEN

Partnering Through the Assessment

Assessment is the pathway for partnering with the family and understanding how to support them. It is generally part of the treatment conceptualization at the beginning of care. To determine the type of support we may provide, we must understand the individuals, the relationships, and the distress they are experiencing. The questions, forms, and collaborations explored at the beginning of care help guide the work. We create hypotheses about etiology and possible treatment interventions as we gather information. Thinking of every conceptualization as a hypothesis helps providers maintain a curious stance. Through curiosity, we can hold that assessment is alive during our work with the family from beginning to end. We are always learning and partnering to discuss our ideas. The deeper the client–provider relationship becomes, the deeper the sharing and understanding. This chapter provides clinicians with a framework for conducting anti-oppressive relationship-based assessments with perinatal families.

REFLECTING ON ASSESSMENTS

The quality of relationships impacts the well-being of all members within a system. When one person in a family is not well, it affects the others. How it impacts them will depend on the specific cultural characteristics of each family and its members. Our capacity to understand the family story rests on building an authentic relationship with the client. An anti-oppressive stance considers the assessment a relational process rather than a set of questions asked at the beginning of treatment. A relational process entails continuity in the partnership

DOI: 10.4324/9781003286394-10

between the assessor and the person being assessed. Systems like insurance companies require information gathering and a medical lens by asking for a diagnosis in the first meeting with the client to reimburse for our services. A Westernized approach to psychotherapy can bypass the slowing down necessary to establish a relationship. We must find ways to navigate this system while honoring non-dominant ways of being (Tenets Initiative, 2018). I aim to support you in developing an anti-oppressive partnership with families. This relational frame invites slowing down the beginning stage of care. In this chapter, you will find questions and ideas to guide your assessment. While the specific tools you choose matter, they are not as critical as your way of being with people. Relationships are the heart of our work and where trust can live. Without trust, we cannot partner to understand the family story. Let us practice some reflection as we think about assessment.

- What thoughts come up for you as you think about assessments?

  _____
  _____
  _____

- How do you prepare yourself for meeting new clients?

  _____
  _____
  _____

- How do you think about relationship building at the beginning of care?

  _____
  _____
  _____

- How long does the beginning of care last?

  _____
  _____
  _____

- How are you creating the therapeutic container as you get to know clients?

  _____
  _____
  _____

- What thoughts come up for you as you think about co-creating the container?

  _____
  _____
  _____

- How are you holding a trauma-informed approach during assessments?

  _____

  _____

  _____

- How has anti-oppressive practice shown up in the way you conduct assessments?

  _____

  _____

  _____

- What barriers are you facing as a provider in applying a relational assessment approach?

  _____

  _____

  _____

BUILDING A COLLABORATION

I invite you to approach the beginning of the work as a place of collaboration and co-creating a container. Anti-oppression is a way of being rather than a set of guidelines to follow (Foronda et al., 2016). Many of us come from backgrounds and training in systematic ways of conducting assessments. We might be used to giving the client a set of questionnaires to answer before the session and a set of forms we complete as part of the clinical interview. The reflections you completed above and in previous chapters serve as a starting point for navigating this work in the context of the U.S. system and society. The U.S. system and society are the context of my experience, which I use to ground this text. I will share some ways of thinking about assessment that you can integrate into your practice. You might have to meditate and reflect with a supervisor on balancing your organization's requirements with this relational way of being. The information I share in this book is a starting point for integrating reflection into your work. I hold the ideal with the reality of the systems, privileges, and barriers we navigate.

In one of my first counseling jobs, some of the insurances accepted by the company allotted a limited number of counseling sessions per client. We had to contact insurance companies to request more units measured in 15-minute increments. Therapists had to demonstrate justification for treatment based on clinical goals and diagnosis. The insurance company often only allotted 12 sessions to work with a family. I felt frustrated because it generally took almost that amount of time to begin feeling welcomed into the family. Providers must earn trust. Trust is not given because we have a degree or the family self-referred to our services. As a recovering perfectionist and newer clinician, I felt I was doing something wrong by not wrapping up treatment at the end of the sessions. My supervisor at the time shared some wisdom with me that I would like to pass on. She said, *"Establishing a relationship is a treatment goal."* It is a simple lesson and vital to centering the client's experience. We can justify care through an anti-oppressive approach. We can protect the therapeutic relationship by slowing down and attuning. We need time to consider the caregiver(s), the child(ren), and the relationship(s) involved. What is happening with each member, and how are they impacting each other? And how is the family experiencing us as the clinician? Speeding up through the beginning stages of care can make us forget our role in the family's dynamic. Slowing down can help us remember that we are balancing supporting and interrupting the family's ecosystem. We are more likely to create unhelpful disruption when we forget to factor our relationship and reflection into our case conceptualization.

One of the first questions I encourage providers to ask is, *"What does the individual or family think is happening?,"* *"How do they understand it?"* This question is our starting point for honoring the client's lived expertise. Putting it into action might mean creating space to name systemic barriers, colonization, intergenerational healing, etc. People may not know precisely why they feel like they do, which is common and okay. We can validate what they share as we listen to their story. Listening and following their need can guide the types of questions we ask the client. I prefer to integrate an organic conversation into my assessment process. My first mental health job was doing biopsychosocial assessment in a mental health community center. The evaluation had multiple pages of questions and checkboxes. It felt instinctual to jump to different queries depending on where the client led me. It never made sense to move question by question, as it makes the flow robotic and disconnected. I start the first session with a prompt similar to *"Can you share more about how you've been feeling lately?"* and move on to understand the client's life and experience. We start with what they think is happening and allow their concerns to lead our time. This way of practicing means that the initial assessment period extends over a few sessions, allowing us to get to know each other. Therapists do not share their personal concerns in sessions, but we share our humanness and how we are, which is as important as what we do (Pawl & St. John, 1998). Authenticity and the therapist's use of self is vital to establishing trust.

I have found that with perinatal clients, providing brief psychoeducation as we are conversing is often helpful. Naming the taboos is a valuable starting point. The taboos are the things we are not supposed to say out loud. Perinatal people are not "supposed" to complain about the hardships of parenthood. Emotional distress during this period often leads to feelings of shame. I might tell a caregiver, *"It is common to have thoughts like I don't think I was made for this, I never really wanted to be a parent, or this was a mistake."* I also share about our society's romanticization of being pregnant and having children (which is very strong in some cultures, including mine). Society sells us an idea that does not exist: Complete joy and fulfillment. We can honor the greatness and gift of caregiverhood while naming the pain. Those two things can co-exist. We can love the children we care for deeply and still need a long break. As we start the assessment process, we are setting the frame for the relationship. I want people to know we can discuss everything that impacts their lives and well-being. It is a simple task. We are naming the obvious: Parenting is hard. However, how many times have you gaslighted yourself throughout your life? We might be used to pushing through the pain without noticing the scars and wounds created. As the person begins to see the pain points, they can continue naming contributors to their feelings. Naming allows the emotion or pain to move from isolation into connection.

The following is an example to bring this section to life.

Amaura is a 31-year-old mother to 18-month-old Alexis and 3-month-old Kai. Her partner is in the military. She is seeking therapy and is reporting symptoms of postpartum depression. In the initial intake phone call, she said, *"I am not myself. I am messing up at every turn."* Amaura arrived a few minutes late to the first assessment session. She reported traffic on her way to leave the children with her partner's mother. After discussing forms and policies, we began the intake.

Therapist: Our time today and during the next three to five meetings will help us get to know each other better and see how I might support you and yours.

Amaura: I hope this can help. I don't know if anything can.

Therapist: You mentioned not being yourself when we spoke on the phone. Tell me more about what is going on.

Amaura: The past months have been tough. This is the worst I've ever felt. I don't want to eat. This is embarrassing, but I don't even want to shower. I still do, but it is hard. I just don't understand. I am tired and angry all the time.

Therapist: [takes a breath] Sounds like you are not feeling like yourself and unsure what's happening.

Amaura: [nods]

Therapist: Caregiverhood is extremely challenging. Way more than we talk about. There are so many pieces to the not feeling like yourself puzzle. Bodies are recovering, we are tired, and everyone demands something of us. I wonder what are some of the puzzle pieces that are adding to not feeling like yourself?

Amaura: I don't know. I mean, I can't sleep or rest.

Therapist: We got a piece here. Not being able to sleep or rest can significantly change how we feel and function. How much sleep are you able to get?

Amaura: A few hours here and there. Last night, Kai went down at three and was back up at six.

[I made a note here to ask about Kai's sleep routine and any concerns we might explore there.]

After understanding Amaura's sleep, I might say, *"We got to sleep as a puzzle piece. What else might be another contributor to how you are feeling?"* However, what the client shares gives me a port of entry to other aspects of their life. For instance, as we get a picture of sleep, the client might share that they were up all night and are scared the baby will stop breathing. My next step in this case will be to validate how scary that feeling must be and to learn more about how it is showing up in their lives. This is an example of the organic conversational process of assessment. One question can lead to another when we attune to what the client is sharing.

We also want to know who they feel might be essential for us to include in the assessment. I prefer to include this conversation in the first session rather than in the consultation call. We have more time to explain and digest information during the first sessions. You might hear a port of entry. In the example above, Amaura mentioned her partner's mother. A loved one might be a vital part of treatment, whether they live in the same or different household from the perinatal person. We want to understand the network of relationships involved in the client's life.

Therapist: Some might find including loved ones in our meetings helpful. You mentioned your partner's mother earlier. I wanted to name this as an option in case she might be of support.

Amaura: Yaniye helps here and there when she can.

Therapist: Having others who can support us here and there can be helpful. It's hard to do it alone and with two small children. As we think about the following weeks in getting to know each other, I want to invite you to think of who might be important to connect with. Perhaps to ask them to one of our meetings or for me to contact them [i.e., other providers].

Amaura: I don't want to stress anyone out with my problems. Yaniye is helpful in an emergency, but she is very nosy, and I know how she feels about mental health.

Therapist: Hmm, sharing with others can be a risk when we need support.

Amaura: I don't even know what I need right now. I hate needing to ask for help. [Cries]

Therapist: [Leans in] It's hard not to feel like ourselves.

Amaura: I'm so angry all the time. I am pushing everyone away.

Therapist: We tend to wrap ourselves for self-protection. Having people come too close when things feel raw is not always safe. Reaching out for support might not exactly look like telling people our full story, and we don't have to invite anyone you do not want into our space.

Amaura: I think maybe my partner. Things are not exactly good at the moment. But I know she is worried about me.

Therapist: We can explore this option in the future. Let's spend some more time on how you are feeling.

In these two session excerpts we have various options to explore: Challenges in the relationship with her partner and Yanine, her capacity to ask and receive support, the children, and what it means for her to see a therapist.

Once we have a sense of what they think is happening and who is essential in their lives, we can explore different ways of moving through the assessment process. We can include formal and informal protocols in the initial assessment process. Standardized tools are available free of charge or for a fee to licensed mental health providers. In a perinatal relationship-based framework, clinicians assess in the context of the gestational caregiver, other caregivers involved, the child(ren), and the quality of their relationships. Chapter 3 briefly discusses three tools for identifying perinatal mental health complications and their limitations: EPDS, GAD-7, and PHQ-9. Formal or standardized tools have been tested on different populations and determined to meet research-based standards for identifying concerns. I will not recommend specific tools for your practice as that is beyond the scope of this book, since most tools have value when paired with a social justice lens. I aim for you to explore how you think about assessment and how to move from directive to relational. It might be helpful to provide information on what to look for in an evaluation. The following section explores the three areas to assess in the clinical interviews: The caregiver, the child, and their relationship. Figure 7.1 shows how each area builds and connects to the other in a circular manner demonstrating the interrelationship.

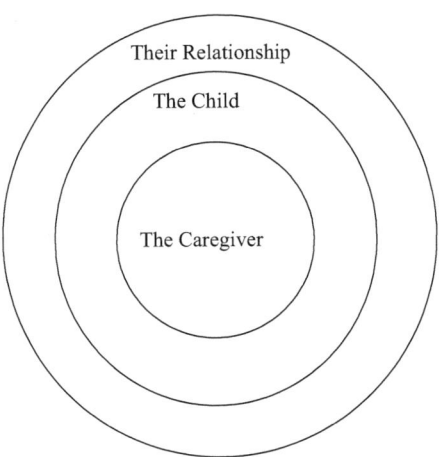

FIGURE 7.1 A Relational Look at Well-Being Between Caregiver and Child

ASSESSING THE CAREGIVER(S)

Consider the life of a caregiver and the different roles they hold. Personal well-being will include the family-of-origin information, culture, mental and physical health history, trauma, significant life events, psychosocial stressors, access to resources, systemic barriers, strengths, and anything else the client might share. Learning about the person's upbringing is vital to an initial understanding of their object relations. As mentioned in Chapter 2, object-relations theory (ORT) is a psychodynamic model which asserts that emotional distress relates to unconscious patterns (Frankland, 2010). People's childhood experiences with their caregivers help form a set of expectations about themselves and the world. We internalize aspects of our caregivers that influence our world and how we perceive communication with others. As assessment is alive throughout treatment, each session will give us more opportunities to collaborate, build, and test hypotheses. However, the beginning stages serve as the initial ground for treatment formulation.

- What parts of their upbringing has the client internalized?
- How have those parts impacted their capacity to care for themselves? A person growing up with an abusive and neglectful parent might be more likely to neglect their needs as an adult (i.e., not listening to their body's cues for hunger, fullness, pain, rest, etc.).
- How does the individual perceive themselves and others?
- How do they perceive their environment, connection to nature, and spirituality?

We want to understand how they care for themselves, receive care, and connect with care. This understanding happens in the context of the micro-(individual), mezzo-(family/environment), and macro-(larger system/society) levels. All levels of questioning are critical to a complete picture of the client, their little one(s), and their relationship(s). Notice how you keep the child(ren) in mind with each question you ask.

We want to understand their feelings, life, object relations, and strengths at the micro-level. In this section of the assessment, we keep a central focus on the person and their internal world.

- How are they feeling emotionally?
- What is important to them?
- What roles do they carry as they navigate their life?
- How is their day-to-day life?
- How was their upbringing?
- What are they concerned about?

- What do they want for themselves?
- What helps them survive when times are tough?

We also want to understand their thoughts about their baby or young child.

- How is the transition to caregiverhood?
- What hopes, dreams, and fears are they holding? In this question, we can tap into their fantasies about becoming a caregiver, such as how they thought they would feel emotionally, the kind of support they imagined they would receive, and how they imagined they would feel about the baby. If there is a gap between the fantasy and the reality, how are they sitting with the discrepancy? Asking about fears the client may have can serve as a port of entry to see if they experience anxiety, intrusive thoughts, panic attacks, or other similar concerns.
- How do they think about their child? The FAN model (See Chapter 5) taps into this concept by asking the caregiver to share three words that describe their child (Gilkerson & Imberger, 2016). Caregivers might struggle to come up with three words for multiple reasons. One of the first is that communicating in single words may not be culturally attuned. Providers can consider asking a question like *"How would you describe your child?"* to explore this idea.

At the mezzo level, we gather information about family, relationships, environment, and community. This set of questions might ask about the quality of relationships with colleagues, their environment, animals, and community involvement. We might ask about the neighborhood, sense of safety, and their capacity to access sunshine and fresh air.

- Who is essential in your life?
- Who is supportive of you?
- Are the relationships you wish were more supportive? In what ways?
- How is life at home?
- How is life outside the home (e.g., work, colleagues, friends, spiritual community, neighborhood)?
- What is it like to be with your loved ones? Our loved ones can be a refreshing breeze after a hot day, providing calm and love. At the other end of the spectrum, they can be the unrelenting sun on a hot day, creating discomfort and possible danger. We might want to go to them for support and instead find judgment or simply the reality that people are busy and we may not be their priority.
- What has shifted in the transition to caregiverhood?
- How is your connection with nature?
- How does spirituality show up in your life?

As we think in a relational context, we also want a sense of how the caregiver imagines this level impacts the child(ren). I encourage providers to listen for themes that might arise. For instance, how is the caregiver holding their child in mind as they share about their life? We might hear their worries, observations of changes, and other projections the caregiver might make. Using our clinical judgment to gauge the client's readiness, we can ask directly, *"How do you imagine this might be for your little one?"* We can hold that question with gentleness and compassion for the caregiver. We can be sure of what we say but not how the other person hears and experiences our words and presence.

At the macro-level, we want to understand access to resources, a sense of safety, barriers, challenges, strengths, culture, and counterculture. We want to bring social determinants of health to the forefront of our work and how we conceptualize distress and psychopathology. As most things in life are interrelated, the questions at the micro-and mezzo-level might give a sense of macro-level issues. For instance, we may get a sense of economic, housing, and interpersonal barriers by asking, *"How is your day-to-day life?"* Here are two ideas to consider:

- How are ancestral, intergenerational, or cultural strengths showing up in your life?
- We can talk about many different things in our work together, including how you are doing financially and how systems like the cost of living, machismo, and racism might impact safety. All is welcome in this space.

When there are other caregivers or adult relationships, we want to know about them and learn from the client how we can integrate them into assessment and care. We are learning from the client because we cannot make assumptions. We want to provide options with a lens of curiosity and humility. In Amaura's excerpt above, the therapist offered a chance for a loved one to accompany the client to a session. The client identified who she wanted to join. An actionable step here for readers is to review your current intake or biopsychosocial assessment forms and notice what you might need to add or ask more about to understand the caregiver within their culture and environment.

ASSESSING THE CHILD(REN)

Please note that diagnosing a young child is unnecessary to provide relationship-based services for perinatal people. An assessment does not need to equal a diagnosis. Our partnering with the caregiver by listening, asking questions, and checking our hypothesis can protect against some harm. However, the reality is that diagnosing comes with labels, stigma, and other barriers, in addition to providing access to the support the family might need. Clinicians integrating the relational approach can consider consulting with other providers or supervisors before diagnosing a young child formally. If you diagnose young children as part of your work, your task will be to consider integrating the caregiver's experience into assessment and treatment.

Children aged 0 to 5 can experience emotional and relational distress. The DC:0–5™ manual can offer a comprehensive way of understanding the child in the context of their environment. Even if you are not diagnosing as part of your practice, I encourage familiarization with this comprehensive way of thinking to help integrate the child(ren) into how you support caregivers. An anti-oppressive lens can support clinicians in considering how systems of power and different forms of oppression impact early childhood. A relational approach to integrating the young child into our work calls for us to hold the caregiver in mind as we understand the child's world. The DC:0–5™ uses an axial system that includes five areas to obtain a comprehensive view for supporting the child: Clinical disorders, relational context, physical and medical health, psychosocial stressors, and developmental context (Zero to Three, 2016). The "organizing framework" for the axial system is a focus on the family and the provider's culture and identity (Noroña et al., 2021, p. 63). The family's culture and expertise and our awareness of the subjective nature of assessments can guide our conceptualization. Although clinical disorder is the first axis in the manual, it needs to be the last aspect explored in our assessment process, as failure to do this can lead to pathologizing developmentally and culturally appropriate behaviors. The manual encourages providers to explore all other areas of a child's life before examining the potential of a clinical diagnosis. A systemic and anti-oppressive approach is a good practice for evaluating individuals and groups across all ages. It can help remind us that no one tool can grasp or meet everyone's needs.

I invite clinicians looking to integrate this manual into their work to think about how they partner with the families in understanding each axis (relational context, physical and medical health, psychosocial stressors, developmental context, and clinical disorders) together. Integrating the baby or young child into the assessment process involves providers collecting data from caregiver interviews, observations, and any formal protocols used. When working with babies and young children, we rely on the caregivers involved to be the holders of the information. Seeing the caregiver as the expert helps us honor non-dominant knowledge and diverse family structures (Tenets Initiative, 2018). Gathering data from caregivers can happen in sessions, phone calls, or forms the caregiver or provider fills out. We want to build a relationship or have a touchpoint with the caregiver/provider when possible. For instance, if the client resides in an intergenerational home, I want to know if the client wants any family members involved, either coming to the session or through a phone call. When a relationship or touchpoint is impossible, especially for providers like teachers or medical doctors who may have limited availability, we can collect information by sending them a tool with the caregiver. This option is imperfect, but we constantly balance the ideal with reality.

Here is an example of an assessment flow using the DC:0–5™ as a guide. Clinical disorders are listed last to highlight the importance of examining all the other factors impacting the child and family.

- Examine the relational context, the quality of the relationships between the child and the caregiver(s), and how the caregivers work together in caretaking (Zero to Three, 2016). The relational context includes how caregivers discipline, allocate duties, support each other, and handle conflict. What and how caregivers share about their children and other adults will help give us a sense of their dynamic. In the case study above, Amaura shared that her partner's mother, Yaniye, was nosy. As the therapist, I want to know what it is like for them to be together. Even if Amaura decides not to include her in our sessions, I will explore how the relationship impacts her well-being and how the children present when they are with her. Children can behave differently across relationships and settings depending on multiple factors. It is possible for people not to get along and still coordinate towards the child's well-being. Ideally, providers can observe interactions between the child and all their primary caregivers in different settings (i.e., clinic, home, childcare). In reality, we might have to think creatively about ways to gather information. Our only option might be to gather information from a third party, as in Amaura's report of the babies' behavior and Yaniye's responsiveness.

  Providers can use structured or unstructured observation models. The ideal situation would be to include both. However, a 30-minute observation at the therapist's office can yield helpful information. The set-up for the observation depends on what is available to each provider. If the observation occurs at your office, have a small area dedicated to the caregiver–child dyad. After explaining the purpose of the observation, you can instruct the caregiver by saying, *"Play with your child as you would if you were alone."* Therapists can observe three components within the relationship: Mutual enjoyment, negotiating stress, and developmentally appropriate expectations.

  Mutual enjoyment can entail characteristics like physical closeness, smiles, laughter, and reciprocity. **Negotiating stress** can show up when a child bids for connection and the caregiver misses it, when the caregiver leads the interaction, and the child is not interested, and when the child feels strong emotions, maybe because they are tired or have difficulty completing a task. Is the caregiver demonstrating **developmentally appropriate expectations**? This component requires the provider to have a basic knowledge of child development and a culturally attuned lens. Is the caregiver demonstrating an expectation that the baby will self-soothe without support? Can the caregiver follow some of the child's lead in interactions?

Clinicians can record observations, when possible, to review with the caregiver or make notes on different moments to discuss. Collaborative observation reviews are vital to ensuring that we partner with the caregiver to understand the meaning of behavior. We can also partner with the client to see how mutual enjoyment, stress negotiation, and developmentally appropriate expectations show up in their caregiving. An intentional conversation around the three components helps us understand what each might mean to the caregiver. For example, mutual enjoyment might involve laughter in one family while sitting quietly by each other in another. Developmentally appropriate expectations vary among different cultural groups, so we want to ensure that the caregiver shares how they understand their child.

- Ask about physical conditions and considerations like events or medications impacting the child (Zero to Three, 2016). Because young children cannot fully communicate their needs, we want to know how this axis might affect observed behaviors. For example, if a child takes a stimulant, how does it impact their clinical presentation? The reports from the childcare provider? The relationship between caregivers and the child? Medical complications can also impact the caregiver's perception of their child. If a child spends six months in the NICU, it will affect relationships, stress, and development for that child and their caregivers. The effect will depend on the multiple factors involved. How does the caregiver perceive their child's vulnerabilities and strengths?

It is also important to mention how critical the provider's reflection is to this process. If the family engages in non-dominant/non-Westernized treatment, how are we partnering with them to understand what is essential? Do we remember that different is not bad or neglectful? How do we obtain support when we do not understand the culture? There is no one correct answer. It is about partnering, listening, and being intentional. Kendi (2019) stated that we move between racist and anti-racist actions throughout life. Being an anti-racist means taking steps that lead to racial equity. What actions are we taking with families that lead to equity?

While working in the early childhood court system, a father I supported tested positive for alcohol during a supervised visitation with their child. I was present at the visit and remember being confused when called into a meeting. We were able to partner with the father to understand what took place. The father explained experiencing a sore throat in the morning and that his mother prepared a home remedy which included rum. We discussed this with the early court team, including the Judge, who still warned the client not to consume alcohol but understood the client's explanation. Our capacity to listen supported our advocacy for the father. In this example, the cause for the child's removal included exposure to cocaine in utero. I share this example because situations are complex and involve "yes and" conditions. What might have occurred for this family with a different team that did not have culture in mind? I imagine one of the possibilities for this father could be for the team to question his explanation and not believe him. Court system teams hold a lot of power over families. We can make recommendations like stopping the supervised visitations, changing or adding mental health and substance use disorder services, parenting classes, and other services that become barriers when not attuned to the family's needs. If we had not believed him, refused to partner with him, and positioned ourselves as the experts, we could have caused some significant harm. Let us imagine that the father then becomes angry at our recommendations in the courtroom. How does his anger at our unjust recommendations impact his case in the long term?

- Ask about psychosocial stressors (Zero to Three, 2016). When assessing, the provider will ask about the family's life experiences. We want to know if the pregnancy, delivery, adoption, or placement were complicated and how long the complications lasted. We collaborate with the family to gain a sense of any stressful or disruptive experiences. Therapists partner with the family to create a narrative of their life and history. Talking about difficult life experiences is another area where we honor that assessment is alive during treatment. People might share more vulnerable material after a period of trust. Introducing families to Adverse Childhood Experiences (ACES) might be a way to gather information in this area. I find it helpful for people to know why I am asking the questions I ask. Giving a rationale for my line of interviews helps us be on the same page. It is also an opportunity to say, *"And if there is something you are not ready to share, that is okay too."*

- Consider that development moves across emotional, social-relational, cognitive, language and communication, and movement/physical domains (Zero to Three, 2016). Children develop incredibly rapidly during the first five years of their life. Each developmental milestone builds on the other. A child who falls outside developmental expectations might experience increased distress, impacting the caregiver–child relationship. For example, a child who needs more support in language development might experience frustration at others for not understanding their needs. Assessing developmental milestones requires using some form of formal tool due to the spectrum of developmental changes across ages. For example, children's social-relational domain will look different at 6 months than at 12 months. It also requires cultural humility in understanding that development and expectations can look different among cultural groups.

  Clinicians can introduce the tool and its purpose to the family, including the types of questions and the possible outcomes. When examining results, we can partner with the family to explore whether it is a concern or if the tool did not pick up on a specific cultural component. Knowing expectations and collaborating can alleviate hesitation. For example, suppose I shared with the caregiver beforehand that we might discuss a referral to another provider, like an occupational therapist. In that case, if there is a concern, it can help ease us into a conversation if the subject comes up.

- Use all the prior information and your anti-oppressive lens (which should be present in everything we do) to explore whether a clinical disorder(s) is present (Zero to Three, 2016). The DC:0–5™ includes a set of mental health conditions deemed applicable to young children. While we know that many clinicians and families have concerns related to diagnosis, like historical harm, the best way to support families is by understanding their needs. When a young child meets the criteria for a clinical disorder, the diagnosis might be the key for the family to access care. One of the issues with clinical conditions is their over-and under-diagnosis. A comprehensive assessment can help providers gather the necessary information to avoid an incorrect diagnosis. Suppose a child brings a diagnosis from another provider. In that case, we must partner with the family and the other provider, when possible, to understand what the child is experiencing. Does the family agree with the diagnosis? Can we coordinate to speak with the provider? Did the provider thoroughly assess the child through an early relational lens? Did the provider consider the family's culture and context? Once conducting the clinical interview and assessment process, do we still agree with the diagnosis? Is further assessment needed from another provider, like an occupational therapist or a neurologist? Does the child need support beyond what we can provide within our discipline and training?

ASSESSING THE RELATIONSHIP(S)

The relational context listed above helps us assess how the caregiver and the child relate and how the adults collaborate to coordinate meeting the child's needs (Zero to Three, 2016). Observations and our conversations give us a sense of the quality of the caregiver–child relationship. We also want to have a sense of how the caregivers relate to others and the quality of those relationships. For example, Amaura and Yaniye might collaborate well towards caregiving but hold discord in their relationships. I worked with a family in two separate households where the coordination for the child was positive, but the adults could not be in the same room. This family communicated only using the court-monitored system and did the parent-to-parent child transition outside of their local fire station. This system worked for them for the three years we worked together. We can argue that if caregivers cannot talk to each other, they cannot negotiate their children's needs, but this might not be true for everyone. In this example, each caregiver recognized what they needed to be present for their child in the context of their relationship. They knew that anything outside of the negotiated lines might have the potential for adverse consequences, and they worked to prevent that from happening. Looking back at the adult dynamics, we see people who cannot support each other.

I want to know if the caregivers can protect themselves. Can they have relationships with the person before them and recognize when expectations are not aligned with reality? For example, Amaura did not think that Yaniye would be supportive. I am interested in knowing if this comes from her experience of Yaniye or past experiences with others now distorting this relationship. Exploration of the meaning of relationships takes time to build. The more we learn about the person, the more we see patterns. We also want to explore what other relationships might be important for the family. For example, how is a connection to the earth impacting the dyad? What about spirituality and aspects like nature, Spirit, high power, or God? Exploring beyond a Eurocentric lens can guide understanding that people have relationships with their environment. These relationships are alive and influence mood, emotional bandwidth, and capacity to give and receive love.

When choosing tools or questions for our clinical interviews, we want to hold the well-being of the caregiver, the child(ren), and the relationship(s).

A NOTE ON FORMAL TOOLS

Administering formal assessments must happen in the context of a relationship. For instance, the Patient Health Questionnaire-9 (PHQ-9) is a tool for identifying depression that we can use in the perinatal period. The tool guides people through symptoms they might have experienced over the past two weeks. Like most resources, the PHQ-9 has some challenges regarding its use across cultures (Harry et al., 2021). For example, it misses some markers of depression among Alaskan and American Indian communities. Clinicians might find it helpful to think of the PHQ-9 and other formal protocols as tools to guide a series of conversations rather than as a one-time protocol. Item two in the PHQ-9 asks about "feeling down, depressed, or hopeless" (Kroenke et al., 1999, para.1). We can introduce the tool as something we will discuss and comment on during our time together. I might explore what it means to feel down for the person. How do they think about depression? How has depression manifested for them or in their community? Maybe we find that the right word for that person is not the medical term but something different. Depression looks different for many of us. In my community, a common term for depression-like symptoms is *malestar*, which loosely translates as overall discomfort. Malestar can include nausea, dizziness, body aches, feeling warm, and many other psychosomatic symptoms that one can experience. Symptoms of malestar can be present in a medical condition like the flu and depression. I will give this example to clients and ask about similar things they, their culture, or their family might describe to indicate an emotional upset.

In this way, we use the PHQ-9 as a tool to guide a conversation rather than as a stand-alone series of questions. You can take any protocol and partner with the client to think about what makes sense regarding the approach. I am thinking of the FAN model and the thinking core process (See Chapter 5). Collaborative exploration (the thinking wedge) is my jam. I enjoy thinking and reflecting with people. The process is slower this way, but I am not sure it was ever meant to be fast. How can I possibly know if someone truly meets the criteria for a disorder if I only had one 50-minute appointment with them? Slowing down is another example where I veer off evidence-based practices. The way I am describing integrating this and other formal tools does not follow its set protocol. I continuously invite clinicians to be attuned to what is happening for them and the client to determine the next steps.

SUMMARY

The greatest success in information gathering is developing a trusting relationship with the client. There is no substitute for partnership and collaboration, which might look different for each family and person. One of the reasons why we consider assessment to be developing throughout the life of treatment is that it takes time to trust. We aim to understand their individual and family functioning as we partner with the client. Reflect on the level of trust it takes to answer explorative questions about our lives and how we might care for our children. In each interaction and disclosure, we might carry the trauma from our current life and the intergenerational pain of our ancestors. Even when people seek treatment of their own accord, it is vital for providers not to take for granted the need to build and earn trust. There is no speeding up of the process of a therapeutic relationship.

REFERENCES

Foronda, C., Baptiste, D. L., Reinholdt, M. M., & Ousman, K. (2016). Cultural humility: A concept analysis. *Journal of Transcultural Nursing: Official Journal of the Transcultural Nursing Society, 27*(3), 210–217. https://doi.org/10.1177/1043 659615592677

Frankland, A. G. (2010). *The little psychotherapy book: Object relations in practice*. Oxford University Press.

Gilkerson, L., & Imberger, J. (2016). Strengthening reflective capacity in skilled home visitors. *Zero to Three, 37*(2), 46–53.

Harry, M. L., Coley, R. Y., Waring, S. C., & Simon, G. E. (2021). Evaluating the cross-cultural measurement invariance of the PHQ-9 between American Indian/Alaska Native adults and diverse racial and ethnic groups. *Journal of Affective Disorders Reports, 4*, 100121. https://doi.org/10.1016/j.jadr.2021.100121

Kendi, I. X. (2019). *How to be an antiracist*. Random House Publishing Group.

Kroenke, K., Spitzer, R. L., & Williams, J. B. W. (1999). Patient Health Questionnaire-9 (PHQ-9) [Database record]. APA PsycTests. https://doi.org/10.1037/t06165-000

Noroña, C. R., Lakatos, P. P., Wise-Kriplani, M., & Williams, M. E. (2021). Critical self-reflection and diversity-informed supervision/consultation: Deepening the DC:0–5 cultural formulation. *Zero to Three, 40*(2), 62–71.

Pawl, J. H., & St. John, M. (1998). How you are is as important as what you do … in making a positive difference for infants, toddlers, and their families. Zero to Three.

Tenets Initiative. (2018). Diversity-informed tenets for work with infants, children & families/Principios informados en la diversidad para trabajar con bebés, niños, niñas y familias. Irving Harris Foundation. https://diversityinformedtenets.org/download-the-tenets/

Zero to Three. (2016). *DC:0–5™: Diagnostic classification of mental health and developmental disorders of infancy and early childhood*. Author.

CHAPTER EIGHT

The Invitation to Deepen the Relationship

Every step we take with a family must consider consent and attunement as vital requirements to navigate their ecosystem without causing harm. Informed consent is an ethical obligation requiring providers to explore the risks and benefits of care to uphold the client's right to self-determination (Trachsel & Holtforth, 2019). Consent involves letting clients know the options available in the counseling process and their outcomes. Discussing possibilities and outcomes allows for thinking together about the next steps in treatment and within each session. Attunement refers to the reflective capacity of a provider to understand what the client might be feeling and experiencing from moment to moment (Gilkerson & Imberger, 2016). Consent and attunement offer a pathway to collaboration and knowing which direction to take. Reflection helps us attune and examine whether a family has provided consent. It keeps us present, flowing, and curious. Reflection is foundational to ensuring we move at the family's pace. I used to think of informed consent as something we did at the beginning of treatment. It involved having clients sign a form that discussed the counseling process, potential benefits, and possible adverse outcomes like the treatment not working. The more I engaged in this work through an anti-oppressive lens, the more I questioned my understanding of collaboration. Consent is not a given at any stage of collaboration. It requires partnership, being in synch with the person, sharing information, and listening. This chapter explores the invitation into treatment through the lens of deepening the clinical relationship.

DOI: 10.4324/9781003286394-11

RELATIONAL HEALTH AND WELL-BEING

Our primary focus is on the well-being of the caregiver, the child, and their relationship. Chapter 7 reviews the steps to assessment leading into conceptualizing initial hypotheses of the family by inquiring at the micro-, mezzo-, and macro-level systems impacting their lives. At the micro-level, we examine the individual constitution of each family member, including risks and protective factors. Next, we look at the family relationships, neighborhoods, schools, and other structures directly and indirectly interacting with them. The macro-level entails systemic barriers like racism, lack of affordable housing, and limited support for undocumented individuals. It is also essential for us as clinicians to examine our capacity to *see* the family's story as they see it and to hold it. Clinicians impact findings and outcomes. Our perceptions, views, and history influence how we understand concerns and strengths. Recognizing this reality is a vital piece of an anti-oppressive framework. Providers are not outside objective viewers. We are active subjective facilitators. We are entering the family's ecosystem and creating changes from the moment we make that first call for a consultation or to schedule an appointment.

The change we bring can be our presence and how we impact the family. For instance, we might be the first person to tell a perinatal caregiver that their pain is real. The changes we create can also be related to how we understand the family's story and the outcomes of that understanding. If a perinatal caregiver shares that they are having intrusive thoughts of stabbing their child and our instinct is to call CPS, we might end up causing harm with an unnecessary call instead of facilitating support. Even if we do not take action on that instinctual response, without reflection, the seed of distrust and the caregiver seen as dangerous is now planted at the heart of the relationship. Another consideration is that our verbal and non-verbal responses give information to the client. A sudden flinch, a shift in our seat, or how we word a question might impact the person's capacity to lean in or out of the relationship. Due to the barriers that racism and colonization create, the potential for adverse outcomes increases with the intersection of marginalized identities. Our presence is an independent variable in conceptualization.

I invite you here to take a moment to reflect on one of your recent new clinical relationships.

- How did your presence impact the treatment conceptualization?

  _____

  _____

  _____

- How did you hold your subjectivity in mind, and how did you communicate it to the family?

_____

_____

_____

Deepening the Relationship

We want to give caregivers an opportunity to discuss and reflect on our initial conceptualizations before exploring readiness to begin treatment. We explore deepening our work with the family after conducting initial assessments and conversations with the family on the findings (see Chapter 7). As we maintain awareness of the continuity of evaluation, attunement, and consent, we can begin to wonder how the family is experiencing our care at each session. In between sessions, families might reflect on and discuss with others how the counseling relationship is going. They might have questions, hesitations, and concerns. How they address concerns depends on many factors, including culture, past trauma, and if they feel *seen* and *heard* by us. This reality might mean that clinicians must invite curiosity about the relationship into each session. Let us look at a case example.

Aneel, pronouns they/them, is a 32-year-old gestational caregiver seeking services for anxiety. They have two children, 8-year-old Umang and 8-month-old Kenali. Aneel reports constant worry about something happening to Kenali. They stated, *"I don't want him out of my sight. When my sister takes him, I am scared she might drop or take him away."* Aneel is experiencing symptoms of perinatal OCD. Aneel planned a home delivery with a queer provider. However, they were diagnosed with pre-eclampsia in their last trimester, requiring an emergency c-section. Aneel reported that their midwife was not allowed into the operating room due to COVID regulations and that they were alone and experienced queer-phobic treatment at the hospital by multiple providers. They reported being "put under" during the c-section and did not meet Kenali until the following day after delivery. Kenali demonstrated some gross motor and socio-emotional delays on the standardized assessments. The therapist observed that Kenali seemed overly excited to meet new people, including reaching out multiple times for the provider to pick him up when Aneel was holding him. When Aneel attempted to hand Kenali to the therapist, they stated, *"You can't stand me, huh?"* to the baby, and they seemed sad. Umang has been struggling in school, and, while she seemed interested in her baby brother, Aneel reported, *"I want Umang to play with Kenali, but he's so little. What if she hurts him or does something to him when I am not looking?"*

After spending five sessions getting to know the family, the therapist discussed concerns about intrusive thoughts, the traumatic birth, and the relationships between family members. They also shared the results of the developmental competency evaluations for Kenali. Aneel was tearful as she heard the concerns. They stated, *"I know this is what I was telling you but hearing it out loud from someone else sounds worse."* The therapist validated and shared that the work entails support and prevention. Aneel reported feeling better about the findings and next steps towards the end of the session.

In today's session, meeting number six, the therapist planned to explore any questions and begin discussing treatment options.

Therapist: We talked about a lot of things last week. I know it was a lot to hear.

Aneel: I can't stop thinking that I am hurting my kids. I am failing.

Therapist: That's a really painful thought. Our minds are so good at self-attacking. Any opportunity it gets, it is ready to jump and destroy.

Aneel: What if it's not my mind? What if it's true?

Therapist: I see a parent who cares deeply about their kids and is doing everything possible to protect them.

Aneel: I am scared it won't get better.

Therapist: You are not sure whether anything will be helpful.

Aneel: What if this doesn't help?

Therapist: When we are in the storm, it feels like it'll never end and won't get better. This is why we are here. To find ways for it to get better.

Aneel: How do we do that?

Therapist: We can talk about some options and see how they sound to you. Then, go from there.

Aneel: Okay.

Therapist: Last week, we talked about a couple of concerns: Scary thoughts that are getting in the way of life, the horrible experience before, during, and after the c-section, and some about Umang and Kenali. Do you have any questions for me now that you have had time to sit with what we talked about?

Aneel: [crying] I was so worried about Kenali and Umang. I am hurting them. I was scared but hoped it wasn't true.

Therapist: [deep breath, leans forward] I see our last meeting left you with a lot of worry and uncertainty rather than hope.

Aneel: It was rough.

Therapist: Thank you for sharing. I see I missed the mark last time. I left you feeling like you were doing something wrong.

Aneel: I know it's your job.

Therapist: Sometimes, I can start offering feedback and suggestions too soon. The feeling of roughness you described can be a sign to slow down a bit.

Aneel: What would that look like?

Therapist: Maybe me listening and understanding more about what you are experiencing and what questions you might have before setting goals and all that.

Aneel: Okay. I am worried about Kenali. Do you think I am really hurting him?

Therapist: That is a really important question. One that I am guessing carries a lot of fear and pain. To answer directly, I do not think you are hurting him.

Aneel: [tearfully] I almost didn't come today. I felt so ashamed.

Therapist: I am glad you are here. I stand by what I said earlier. I see a parent who cares deeply about their children. Would it be helpful to talk a bit more about your concerns?

Aneel: Yes, I was so worried about him not sitting on his own. I was trying to watch him this week and realized he doesn't spend time on the floor. I am always carrying him.

In this excerpt, the therapist revisits the previous session to explore questions the client might have. You might notice misattunement right at the beginning of the session. The client shares the concern, and the therapist is working to instill hope before leaning into validation and curiosity by stating, "*I see a parent who cares deeply about their children and is doing everything possible to protect them.*" I included it in this excerpt, as the goal of our work is not perfection. There will be moments of misattunement. We want to ensure the client is leading the session and that we move at their pace. Everything the client shares with us is a gift about their needs and how we might proceed. When we move too fast, we can use the client's response as a guide to re-attune. We see a mismatch in the prior session where the therapist may have moved too quickly with their findings and hypothesis. The therapist worked to create space for bringing Aneel's concerns, recognizing rupture, and creating space for repair. The therapist's capacity to reflect on moving the session too fast is an example of Tenets "Self-awareness leads to better services for families" and "Understand that language can hurt or heal" (Tenets Initiative, 2018, para. 1, 6). In this example, the therapist used language to celebrate the parent's care for their children, causing a rupture. Aneel leaned into the process and named their fears and worries. The rest of the session focused on discussing strengths as a pathway to deepening the work.

An invitation suggests an openness to choices. The client can lean in, lean out, or stand still. When we lean into the counseling relationship, we move towards openness in sharing (verbal and non-verbal). Leaning out might entail a reaction of our nervous system towards self-protection. When things move too fast, too soon, our brains help us survive. In the leaning out, one can leave the counseling relationship by not returning to services or putting up a self-preserving wall (conscious or unconscious). How the barricade shows up will depend on each individual. Some individuals might start to forget sessions, arrive late, or not take conversations deeper. Standing still is also complex to figure out. It could be like putting up a temporary wall while we wait and see if it is safe to take it down. Aneel reported that they almost did not attend the session. Without repair, Aneel might choose to end therapy. I might share this process of leaning in, out, or standing still with clients and explore where they might be at each point in our collaboration. As the provider, the more we lean in, the more likely the person is to partner with us. Of course, in everything we do, we must consider reflection, anti-racism, anti-oppression, and goodness of fit. For instance, when a client misses a session or arrives late, therapists can be curious whether this is a response to something from a previous session or a result of a barrier, like needing to work multiple jobs, high stress, or limited transportation when hosting in-person appointments.

At the end of the last session, Aneel and the therapist decided to continue working together. For the seventh session, Aneel reports feeling more hopeful.

Therapist: It is good to reconnect. How was it for you to be in your life this past week?

Aneel: I made it another day.

Therapist: Yes. That is worth noting. You are still here.

Aneel: I am tired of feeling like this.

Therapist: It's been a rough nine to ten months.

Aneel: Will it ever be better?

Therapist: With the right support, some things can get better. That's why we're here to figure out the right support for you. We can focus on that some more today.

Aneel: I don't know if I can feel better. I've been thinking a lot about my mom. How checked out she was. That's not what I want for my kids.

Therapist: You want something different for your kids. We've been having a lot of conversations that stir up the past.

Aneel: You can say that again.

Therapist: You want to give them a different experience than the one you had.

Aneel: I'm just constantly worried that I am not good enough.

Therapist: This is part of our work together. Noticing the inner narrator who says we are not good enough and how it gets in the way of how we feel.

Aneel: I had this moment where I just wanted to run away and leave it all behind.

Therapist: A painful and relatable moment of parenthood.

Aneel: What do you mean?

Therapist: It's one of those taboos I mentioned during our first meeting. We are not supposed to say that parenting is excruciatingly difficult. That we can love our kids and desperately need a break.

Aneel: I feel like I am the only one.

Therapist: It can feel that way. There are a lot of things that we don't tend to talk about as a society. The pain that comes with parenting is one of those.

Aneel: We need to talk more about it.

Therapist: Mm-hmm, can you share more about what happened when you wanted to run away?

Aneel: Kenali has been wanting to get into everything. I don't want him to put things in his mouth or to get hurt. He wanted to play with Umang, but I had to be in the kitchen.

Therapist: He wants to explore more, which can increase the volume of anxiety. Does that sound right?

Aneel: Yeah, he wants to do everything on his own, and I can't just leave him alone.

Therapist: Hmm, it's interesting your mind went all the way to leaving him alone.

Aneel: I am scared of letting my guard down. He wants to be on the move. I don't know how to be okay with it and keep him safe.

Therapist: I wonder if you would like to work on this together. Looking at how Kenali's need for exploration impacts anxiety and vice versa.

Collaboration also entails balancing creating measurable goals and genuinely connecting with a family. Aneel is letting us know they are ready, and treatment must move slowly. By this stage, the therapist has formulated some hypotheses about the distress. One is that Kenali's push towards exploration increases Aneel's anxiety. Each conversation and information the caregiver shares helps us test our theories. We want to listen to everything the client says verbally and non-verbally as a possible port of entry. A psychodynamic framework lets us recognize that everything shared (and sometimes not shared) in session has meaning (Frankland, 2010). We listen to examine how deeply we can move into each subject.

When Aneel shared about their mom, the therapist had to validate it while keeping in mind the current developmental stage of the therapeutic relationship. The clinical relationship is in its early stages, meaning that the depth of connections and interpretations must match this initial period. Attuning to the clinical relationship helps providers gauge whether we need to seek consent before moving forward. Consent does not need to be fancy. It can be as simple as asking, *"What do you think?"* or *"How does that sound?"* The tricky piece of consent is that the therapeutic relationship is not balanced and equally dynamic. The therapist holds power. Clients might feel that they have to respond positively. Sometimes, the therapist might be able to notice a discrepancy between the client's agreement to proceed and their affect or other non-verbal communication. Seeing contradiction can be a port of entry to explore concerns and to name that not agreeing with the therapist is allowed in the space we are co-creating. Other times, when the client is still unsure of our suggestion, we might misread the discrepancy, not notice it, or it might be invisible altogether. A tip to build collaborative clinical relationships is to invite the possibility of different opinions and to make decisions together. The consistency in how we show up, the questions we ask, and our openness contribute to building trust.

Therapist: It looks like we have a starting point for working together.
Aneel: My anxiety and Kenali?
Therapist: And how anxiety impacts parenting and you as an individual. How does that sound?
Aneel: Okay. How do we do that?

Aneel and the therapist have established a goal and are ready to consider the next steps. Please take a moment here to stop and reflect on these questions:

- How was it for you to read through this excerpt?

  _____
  _____
  _____

- What did you imagine this was like for Aneel and the therapist?

  _____
  _____
  _____

- What questions do you have about Aneel and the therapist?

  _____
  _____
  _____

- What would you have done differently?

  _____
  _____
  _____

- What do you notice about yourself as you reflect on these questions and the excerpt?

  _____
  _____
  _____

- What would it be like to think of everything we do as an invitation and everything the client shares as a gift to the relationship?

  _____
  _____
  _____

DEVELOPING A SESSION STRUCTURE

The structure and frequency of sessions depend on individual needs, availability, and emotional capacity. It might be helpful at the beginning to meet weekly, giving an opportunity to build a relationship and consistency. Sometimes, we might complete an assessment and notice that the person would benefit from meeting twice weekly. However, the capacity to meet often and regularly depends on availability, access, and bandwidth. Families with young children often experience high stress levels and limited capacity for new tasks, making meeting twice weekly tricky and sometimes impossible. The stress and limited capacity of early caregiverhood are other reasons I vouch for combining perinatal and early relational services. We want to hold the ideal and realistic in mind as we collaborate with families. When making decisions together, naming the space between the perfect and practical is helpful. I might say, *"It looks like meeting twice weekly might be beneficial. This frequency would be ideal to start. Now, the ideal and the realistic are not always in line. What meeting frequency would be realistic for you and your family?"* This step also helps test the hypothesis about what I, as the therapist, feel is realistic for the individual. It helps me escape the unintentional mind-frame of making decisions for people.

The Tenet "Work to acknowledge privilege and combat discrimination" can guide us in noticing the subtle ways we might make decisions for people (Tenets Initiative, 2018, para. 3). What we have access to, meaning our privilege, informs our decision-making. Privilege can be as invisible to us as the air we breathe. We can honor that there needs to be continuity to build a relationship. At the same time, can we see how classism, for example, might show up in the expectation to meet once weekly? What about ableism? Best practices are only *best* if they meet the family's individualized needs.

Will it be easier for me to develop a relationship with a family if I can meet with the family weekly? The answer is: Probably so. The first thing that comes to mind is that flexible session frequency challenges my training and what I believe works best. I worry about having a schedule that makes sense for me as a provider and that I may not be as effective without consistency. I think about the capitalist systems we navigate. For clinicians in private practice, regularity and consistency also mean our capacity to pay our bills, save for retirement, and to care for those we love. Providers working for organizations may also have imposed expectations to meet a certain number of clinical hours per week, limiting capacity to offer unlimited flexibility. Organizations face the challenge that inconsistent billing practices can impact the money that comes in and the livelihood of the company and its employees. In this reflection, we as providers also hold the ideal and the reality of our lives. First, notice what makes sense for you as a provider. Second, question the lens you bring and how you can find ways to partner with the family.

The Provider as an Active Component to Determining Session Structure

Let us engage in some reflection about our role in determining session structure. We, as providers, are in the equation. Our thoughts, needs, identities, privileges, and all of who we are are vital to decision-making. If I offer an option that goes against my needs, I run into the danger of regretting it. If I am aware and able to work through the regret, I might be able to realign the balance between me and the client's needs. Without awareness, I may risk holding resentment against the client. I may start to feel uncomfortable before a session, forget our scheduled time, or demonstrate my resentment in other ways. I once had a provider who met me with a sliding scale fee and began shortening the length of our session time. We started with 50-minute appointments, and by the end of the relationship a few months later we were ending at the 36-minute mark. I do not know if resentment was a part of why the provider shortened our sessions. However, I do know that I felt unwanted and unimportant. When we are not reflective and aligned with our needs as providers, we increase the potential to harm the clinical relationship and the client. No perfect answer to this journey will meet everyone's needs. My invitation is to explore what works for you, to hold the reality of you as a human therapist, with needs and desires, serving another human with their own needs and wishes. The more I can see my need and desire, the better I can see it in others.

- How do you make decisions about treatment frequency?

  _____
  _____
  _____

- What do you need as a provider?

  _____
  _____
  _____

- How do you work best?

  _____
  _____
  _____

- What do you like your schedule to look like?

  _____
  _____
  _____

- How do these answers align with the individual needs of the families you serve?

    o   If parts are out of alignment, what must you do to re-attune?

    _____

    _____

    _____

- Why is this important?

    _____

    _____

    _____

Therapists are not blank slates. We have our internal object relations, history, and barriers. Remember that who we are is within us in every space we are in. I cannot check out my needs at the door. The best I can do is to be aware of a need within me. With awareness of my needs, I can prevent projecting them into the client. As you clarify what makes sense, you can hold the container for the clinical relationship. The container is the frame: Frequency of meetings, session length, start/end times, location, and who is welcomed into the space. We aim to continuously bring self-awareness to the forefront of our work with families (Tenets Initiative, 2018).

THE CONTAINER

In Eduardo Duran's keynote speech at the Zero to Three Learn Institute in December 2022, he called for practitioners to bring sacredness into counseling. The therapeutic container is one of the places to hold that sacredness. Duran's book, *Healing the soul wound: A trauma-informed counseling for indigenous communities* (2019), offers a framework for moving away from dominant practice paradigms. One lesson (among so many) from his book is to treat counseling sessions as ceremonies. As one of the many daughters of the Latin American & Caribbean diaspora (Venezuela, Colombia, and Cuba), I have several things that mean ceremony to me. Notice what comes up for you as you think about ceremony. There might be things that automatically come to mind that help you ground before you begin a session, such as taking a quiet moment or deep breaths. I also hold space for the reality that some of us might have a conflictive relationship with the word *ceremony*. One place people go to when they think of the word *ceremony*, especially those of us holding non-Indigenous identities, might be religious trauma. If that is where your body, mind, or heart went, I invite you to reflect on what you notice. See if there is a way to make peace with either the word or the idea of the ceremony. You may call your grounding time something different, which is okay. The key is to find a rhythm that helps you transition into the counseling space and honor the importance of your time together.

Holding deep respect for our work can help us bring our whole-selves into the session. FAN, one of my favorite models for attunement, outlines five core processes that allow providers to listen deeply and focus on the client's lead (Heller & Breuer, 2015). The processes are mindful self-regulation, empathic inquiry, collaborative exploration, capacity building, and integration (See Chapter 5). Mindful self-regulation is the calming step. It refers to what the provider does to prepare themselves emotionally for each meeting with a client and how they remain attentive to their internal world throughout the session. The calming wedge can allow providers to bring a sense of ceremony into their work. Attention to our inner world and its calming is something that we must do throughout all phases of our partnering with people.

Systems and societal discourses impact how we navigate relationships, including psychotherapy. For instance, capitalism connects human worth to productivity (Oluo, 2022). Hustle culture is a product of capitalism that pushes us to move through tasks without pausing to reflect on what it is like to be with ourselves and others. In counseling, therapists can place and experience outside pressure from supervisees and payees on the need to reach specific therapeutic goals. Our need "to be effective" can pollute our capacity to attune to the client. Internal regulation is a skill that can help providers slow down. By slowing down, we can ensure we move at the individual's pace.

I have short legs, and often, when I am on a walk with others, I find myself needing to speed up my stride to keep up. My breath speeds up, and I might lose track of what the other person says. With practice, I am now better at saying, *"Hey, I need to slow down,"* but this was not always the case. Sometimes, we can find ourselves being that person with the longer strides who is not noticing that the other person is panting and left behind. It is never done out of malice but rather because our experience informs our perspective. In this scenario, especially at the beginning of care, the therapist is responsible for ensuring attunement. Mindful self-regulation is slowing down and checking that the pace is comfortable for the other.

Here are some options for ceremony activities that providers can do before a session or to mark the beginning of the meeting with clients.

Tools to Creating Ceremony

- Anoint yourself with oil.
- Cleanse your office (smoke or sound).
- Dance to lively music.
- Light incense or a candle.

- Listen to some words of inspiration.
- Make a cup of tea and take five minutes to notice its smell and warmth.
- Meditate.
- Pray.
- Pull a card on behalf of the client (many decks to choose from).
- Read a poem.
- Stretch your body.
- Take three deep breaths.
- Use visualization.

Therapist: Now that we have a loose plan, how do you feel talking about our meeting frequency?

Aneel: I feel better about starting.

Therapist: I am glad. I am feeling better, too. Thank you so much for sharing and being in this with me. I usually find that having a set appointment time helps us maintain consistency. In our phone call you mentioned your schedule changes a lot, and it might be hard to do this.

Aneel: I've been working from home, which is so good, but being in meetings with Kenali is hard. My boss changes things around often. Sometimes, I think I have a free hour, and something comes up at the last minute.

Therapist: I imagine this is one of those contributors to stress.

Aneel: Yeah, things have been getting worse at work.

Therapist: I can offer some options and would love to hear what you think and if you have other ideas that might work better for your family.

Aneel: You still can't see us on a Sunday, huh?

Therapist: That would make things easier, but I am still out of the office on the weekend.

Aneel: I know. I just wanted to check, just in case.

Therapist: What has been most helpful to you in scheduling our first meetings so far?

Aneel: I had a few days off, which helped. Being able to have Kenali in our meetings. I don't have to worry about leaving him behind.

Therapist: So, morning appointments while Umang is in school might work.

Aneel: I also liked that we've been meeting online. I don't have to worry about being away from work for long. But we also had to cancel one of the appointments.

Therapist: Yeah, and we made it work. We can schedule a standing morning appointment or try week by week. One downside is that meetings will depend on my availability. I will try to hold a morning appointment, but there might be weeks when I can't.

Aneel: Week by week is better because I can try to block out time around meetings and stuff.

Therapist: Great. Let's plan for that. How would this coming Tuesday at 10 a.m. work for you?

Aneel: That works. How long do we meet?

Therapist: I schedule meetings at 50 minutes. I will wait 15 minutes for you if I don't hear from you. If you are running late, message me, and I can wait. However, we probably won't be able to extend our time for that session, so we will have as much time as there is left. How does that sound?

Aneel: I wish I had more time than the 50 minutes, but I know that is hard.

Therapist: One thing we can think about is meeting twice weekly. Meeting more often can be good and bad. The good is more collaboration, and the bad is additional strain on your time.

Aneel: I don't have it in me to take another day of the week for therapy.

Therapist: This is another example of the ideal versus the realistic. What really will work best is what's realistic for you and your family, and we can honor that in our space.

In Aneel's example, you see flexibility in scheduling held within boundaries. The therapist collaborates in developing a plan and naming the wish to meet more often while honoring the client's needs.

As the therapist in this scenario, I want to open my Sunday to meet their needs. However, if I do that I will feel frustrated at having to log in for a session on my day off. I also know, unfortunately, from experience, that I will hold more resentment if Aneel misses a session. The yucky parts of me will get stirred up, and I feel angry that *I came into work on my day off, and they did not bother to show up.* That is my human therapist reality. This example does not mean that opening up a day off or working later to meet a client's needs would be wrong. Therapists must reflect on their why and how they genuinely feel about it. If I can work through my frustration, serving the client on a Sunday is ideal. But if I cannot or do not want to, then there is a high likelihood that my frustration will taint the relationship. Clients do not owe us anything, even when we overextend ourselves. When I start to feel that the client owes me, that is my clue that I am stepping away from my value system. In this journey of being anti-oppressive, we can't forget ourselves. What we think and want is part of the equation.

SUMMARY

Moving the clinical relationship from assessment to treatment requires collaboration. Clinicians can use attunement to ensure we move at the client's pace.

Slowing down in session entails awareness of our internal processes, including needs and desires. When we bring the idea of ceremony into our space with clients, we create a pathway for connection. To connect with the other, we must connect with ourselves first. Self-awareness helps us decrease the potential of harm within the clinical relationship. It is a way to honor our subjectivity and how we impact assessment and treatment outcomes. The more we lean into our internal process, the more we align with the client.

REFERENCES

Duran, E. (2019). *Healing the soul wound: A trauma-informed counseling for indigenous communities*. Teacher's College Press.

Frankland, A. G. (2010). *The little psychotherapy book: Object relations in practice*. Oxford University Press.

Gilkerson, L., & Imberger, J. (2016). Strengthening reflective capacity in skilled home visitors. *Zero to Three*, 37(2), 46–53.

Heller, S. S., & Breuer, A. (2015). Fussy baby network New Orleans and Gulf Coast: Using FAN to support families. *Zero to Three, (35)*3, 56–62.

Oluo, I. (2022, January 6). Capitalism sucks, but don't be shamed for your hustle. https://ijeomaoluo.substack.com/p/capitalism-sucks-but-dont-be-shamed

Tenets Initiative. (2018). Diversity-informed tenets for work with infants, children & families/Principios informados en la diversidad para trabajar con bebés, niños, niñas y familias. Irving Harris Foundation. https://diversityinformedtenets.org/download-the-tenets/

Trachsel, M., & Holtforth, M. G. (2019). How to strengthen patients' meaning response by an ethical informed consent in psychotherapy. *Frontiers in Psychology*, *10*(1747), 1–6. https://doi.org/10.3389/fpsyg.2019.01747

Interventions for Perinatal Individuals and Their Little Ones

CHAPTER NINE

Parental Reflective Capacity

As therapists, building relationships requires self-awareness. The more I under-stand my feelings, thoughts, and desires, the more I can be present for others. Awareness of my internal world allows me to attune to others. When we enter the treatment space with a family, we begin to attune to each individual's needs. Being with the caregiver entails my capacity to *see* them and myself. The thera-peutic *seeing* of the caregiver is a bridge for the caregiver to *see* themselves and their child. Parental reflective functioning refers to the caregiver's capacity to recognize their child's internal world while being aware of their inner experiences and how interactions with their child impact them (Luyten et al., 2017). This chapter explores how therapists can support caregivers' reflective capacity to effect long-lasting changes in the family system.

REFLECTIVE CAPACITY AND SENSITIVITY

Luyten et al. (2017) explain that reflective functioning, also known as mentalizing, is one's "capacity to think and feel about thinking and feeling, to look at oneself from the outside and at others from the inside" (p. 175). I think about it as creating a bridge into the other person's world. The fact that there is a bridge helps me remember that I have a whole world inside me. Self-awareness, the starting point for The Tenets, is the compass to finding our way to others (Tenets Initiative, 2018). The compass has to come with me when I attempt to enter another person's world. It helps me attune and know how to proceed with each step. Parental reflective functioning, which I will refer to as caregiver reflective functioning (CRF),

DOI: 10.4324/9781003286394-13

is the pathway to sensitive and responsive caregiving (Madsen et al., 2023). Sensitive caregiving accurately interprets the needs of the child more times than not. It entails the caregiver having emotional awareness, meaning being able to know how they are feeling. When a toddler is experiencing a meltdown, the caregiver must recognize and soothe their frustration to respond appropriately to the child's needs. It is being able to say to ourselves as adults, "*This moment is difficult.*" Then, we can give ourselves what we need to calm distress and be present for the other. When caregivers can validate the moment's difficulty for themselves, it can open up space for seeing the child.

Recognizing our dysregulation helps us remember that young children cannot regulate their distress. It can help us see how we may respond to the child. Is the caregiver unintentionally yelling, raising their voice, or putting it on the child to regulate themselves? An accurate understanding of how a child feels is a map to responding in a way that meets their needs. The goal is never perfection. There will be times when caregivers misread an interaction and others when we, as clinicians, misinterpret them. Misattunement is part of life. When a mismatch happens, we seek to repair it. Repair is key. It demonstrates empathy and connection. The essence of reflective functioning is noticing when we respond in a way that missed the mark and making an attempt to reconnect. A caregiver who sees a rupture holds their child's experience in mind (Slade, 2005). They are putting words, emotions, and thoughts into their child's inner world in a way that aligns with what the child is actually feeling and experiencing.

CALEB AND YURISBEL'S STORY

Caleb was 23 months old when his adoptive mom, Yurisbel, brought him in to counseling. Yurisbel was concerned about Caleb's behaviors during transitions, like bedtime and getting ready for daycare in the morning. She explained that she was trying to potty train him but felt he *"did not listen"* and was *"being confrontational to get his way."* I wondered about Caleb's readiness to begin potty training and what their interactions were like at home. Yurisbel understood the challenges in potty training to mean that Caleb was being purposefully difficult. Her verbalizations helped me create some hypotheses about her reflective capacity. Could she see the world through Caleb's eyes? Was there a power struggle due to expectations beyond Caleb's current capacity? How aware was she of her emotional state when interacting with her child? How was her behavior impacting Caleb, and could she see that impact? I frame my hypothesis as questions as a reminder to remain curious.

Yurisbel adopted Caleb when he was 18 months old after a year of being his foster parent. She reported that the adoption process was emotionally distressing, as there were several times when she did not know whether Caleb would return to his biological parents. She thought that the finalization of the adoption would bring joy. Instead, she found herself experiencing sadness, feelings of emptiness, and fearing that Caleb would get hurt and be taken away. She expressed shame at the increased anxiety, stating, *"This is what I wanted. I should feel grateful."* Therapists can use the clinical relationship to increase CRF. Perinatal caregivers face shame and isolation when they are not wearing the mask of joy. Wearing the mask can mean pretending things are alright to others or saying that we do not need support when we desperately need it. When a child joins a family, mental health complications are not limited to biological caregivers. Complications affect gestational and non-gestational caregivers (Mental Health America, n.d.; Postpartum Support International, n.d.). The adjustment, changes, and flooding of emotions following heightened anxiety can trigger symptoms of depression and anxiety. These possible changes to the mental health and well-being of an adoptive caregiver can be easily overlooked by providers.

Yurisbel and Caleb participated in counseling with me for two years. Sessions entailed a combination of dyadic (caregiver–child) and individual sessions (caregiver only). The dyadic sessions offered an opportunity to enhance their relationship, while the individual sessions with the caregiver provided a private space to freely process painful memories and thoughts. Yurisbel shared that when she was 5 years old, her mother and some family members made plans to travel from Cuba to Miami in a *balsa* (raft/small boat). Her mother drowned during the journey, and she was raised by her maternal aunt. Observations of interactions with the dyad revealed that Yurisbel seemed hypervigilant of Caleb's behavior. She followed him around, cleaning up after everything he touched, and wanted him to play right in front of her without exploring the room. The more I learned about Yurisbel's history, the more I began to connect how parenthood was triggering her past trauma (Fraiberg et al., 1975). Selma Fraiberg introduced the term *ghosts in the nursery* to represent unremembered parts of a caregiver's past that negatively affect caregiver–child relationships. The loss of Yurisbel's mother and the distress of the adoption process were present in every interaction between her and Caleb. Her fear that Caleb would be taken away or that something might happen to him may be a remanent of the loss of her mother. I wondered if she was ready to begin working on reflective capacity or whether we needed to slow down and create space for attunement into her internal world and grief. How many experiences of being seen and heard did she have in her life? Was she attuned to the impact of the traumatic loss of her mother in her life? The survival tendency to dissociate from pain by getting up, dusting off, and continuing each time we fall can blur our awareness of trauma's presence.

LOOKING AT THE PARALLEL PROCESS

To support Yurisbel's reflective capacity, I had to attune to my own. I felt a sense of compassion and sadness as I heard her story of losing her mother so tragically and so young. My own psychotherapy and reflective supervision are a crucial part of my work. As much psychotherapeutic processing as I have done, pieces of my childhood trauma still get stirred up. Awareness of my feelings and thoughts allowed me to soothe internal discomfort and create space for holding Yurisbel's pain and tolerating some of her mismatches with Caleb. I am unsure if the word *tolerating* is the best descriptor for my internal journey. I am using the term *tolerate* to describe my need to slow down and move out of the role of the expert. I needed to understand and partner with the dyad before moving into action and giving tools. Before imparting my judgment, I wanted to understand what the behavior meant to the caregiver. I am Latina and trained in a dominant and Eurocentric way. Seeing my feelings and initial interpretations of their interactions was crucial to partnering. Judgment does not encourage relational growth. Promoting lasting change in counseling relies greatly on the clinical relationship. My anti-oppressive lens helps me move out of the need to "fix" into follow the family's needs.

An internal concern that often arises for me is *"Am I enough?,"* *"Is this enough?"* This fear often parallels the struggles and internal dialogue of caregivers. The caregiver and I are walking a journey of support. Partnering with her helps her partner with her child. The parallel process refers to my capacity as a provider to positively influence the caregiver's relationship with their child (Stroud & Morgan, 2014). The influence takes place as I model sensitivity and responsiveness. In a way, we can say that experiencing someone's reflective capacity is vital to developing our own. This concept is strongly linked to the interlocking relationship between supervisor–practitioner, practitioner–caregiver, and caregiver–child (Heffron & Murch, 2010). Check out Chapter 5 to learn more about the parallel process in reflective supervision/consultation.

As clinicians, we often have to weigh the balance of allowing the family to lead while ensuring the child's safety. One of the issues I have run into in my practice and consulting with clinicians is how we define safety. When we decide to bridge a family or caregiver into a specific intervention, are we doing so out of our uncertainty or out of a need displayed by the family? For example, when Yurisbel redirects Caleb to stay close to her during our meeting at my office, my first instinct is to say, *"Hmm, I wonder if it might be okay for him to look around. I have a lot of cool toys here that he might like."* If I make that comment without understanding their dynamic, I may undermine Yurisbel's role or push her into doing something that she is uncomfortable with. The idea here is for clinicians to remain curious about what is happening from moment to moment before giving guidance. I invite you to pause here to reflect on these questions:

- How do you define safety as it relates to the clinical space?

  _____
  _____
  _____

- What situations are appropriate to sit back and be curious?

  _____
  _____
  _____

- Which instances would you remain curious about while stepping in and redirecting?

  _____
  _____
  _____

- How are you tracking your reflective capacity and using it to build CRF?

  _____
  _____
  _____

SESSION EXCERPT FROM CALEB AND YURISBEL

The beginning of our work focused on learning about Yurisbel's story. As she reflected on her story, Yurisbel began to acknowledge the impact of her early childhood losses on who she is and how she parents. The more Yurisbel recognized her internal world, the more she began to *see* Caleb. Distressing mental health symptoms decreased, and dyadic relationships strengthened. I will share an excerpt from one of our sessions about six months into our collaboration:

Therapist: How has it been like for you to be Caleb's mother since we last met?
Yurisbel: It's been a heavy week. Some days, we are working well, and I feel good; other days, he is pushing me away.
Therapist: hmm ...
Yurisbel: I know he gets overwhelmed with changes but giving him what he needs is hard. I wish it were easier.
Therapist: When he gets upset, he gets upset. It is a hard ask to stay calm with a screaming toddler.
Yurisbel: I feel so helpless. I want him to stop and do what I am asking. It was so simple this week. He sat on the potty for a while and then, 20 minutes later, peed his pants. I almost lost it.
Therapist: Potty training has been very hard for both of you.

145

Yurisbel: I guess it's hard for him too. I was so mad, and I looked at him, and he looked so scared of me. He didn't even cry. It was like he was in shock.

Therapist: Looks like you noticed something in him even when he wasn't sharing it with words.

Yurisbel: I hadn't realized he could get so scared of me. I thought, "I can't do this." Maybe potty training needs to stop for a bit.

Therapist: What would it be like for things to pause for a bit?

Yurisbel: We would have some peace and one less thing to fight about. I want him to be excited about potty training. For us to connect and high-five instead of him being scared and me feeling angry. Maybe if we do it later when he's ready, it will be smoother.

Therapist: That's an experiment worth trying, and you both need some peace in your lives after so much has happened. Checking for his readiness seems like a great idea.

Yurisbel: I wanted to feel like we were starting new, and this felt like something I could do as his mother. As his real mother, finally.

Therapist: [Takes a deep breath] This was about much more than potty training then.

Yurisbel: I guess. It was something we could do as a new chapter of our family.

Therapist: A starting-together ritual.

Yurisbel: Kinda, we had to report on everything we did. I was so ready for it all to be over and start anew. To prove to myself that we could do it. That I can do this one thing for him on my own.

Therapist: hmm, sounds like a lot of pressure on you and him after a very stressful period, especially since potty training requires both of you to be in it and ready.

Yurisbel: I hadn't thought much about his stress. I think I need to slow down for many reasons, not just my frustration, but he has been through a lot in the past year.

In this excerpt we can see how Yurisbel became aware of her emotional state and noticed when Caleb felt afraid. Not only was she able to notice that he was scared but she connected it to her reaction to him. She saw the impact of her behavior on Caleb. She saw that his fear was not defiance and that the issue was not him "not listening" but was about his readiness and her reaction. In turn, she was able to think of a different way of moving forward that honored both of their needs. Potty training is challenging for many caregivers. However, as we build CRF, we must explore what each specific experience or activity means for the caregiver. For Yurisbel, potty training was a chance to experience herself as Caleb's mother without the eyes of the Court system on her. She wanted to prove to herself that she could raise him, that she was a good mother. When things did not move smoothly, it began impacting her insecurities related to her grief and the trauma of the adoption process. Once we got to the deeper meaning of potty training, Yurisbel could see that it was not about Caleb but rather about proving something to herself. She could see the stress she was putting on Caleb and herself to perform. In letting go of the expectation of perfect timing around this developmental task, she could stop judging herself for "failing" and recognize Caleb's needs. She was also able to identify the impact of the adoption process on Caleb's emotional well-being.

Understanding their potty-training journey was our pathway to Yurisbel responding in more attuned ways to other behaviors. In bridging Caleb's world, she began to wonder about other cases where she used to think of him as confrontational. For example, she began supporting his challenges with transitions from task to task by implementing small changes, like giving him a warning instead of trying to pick him up to move him to another room or activity. Individual sessions served as a space for her to process traumatic memories and to understand her internal world. She explored her relationship with her aunt growing up, which, although close, did not allow for conversations about the loss of her mother. She was able to hold kindness for herself. The more presence she extended to her story, the more emotionally present she was for Caleb.

WATCH, WAIT, AND WONDER

I was also interested in creating space to address some hypervigilance observed during the assessment and subsequent sessions. Watch, wait, and wonder (WWW) is a strategy that supports caregivers in shifting from directive interactions to following their child's lead (Cohen et al., 1999). This tool can aid caregivers in attuning to their children while exploring their internal representations. The instructions for this intervention are reflected in its name. Muir (1992, p. 321) explained:

> The technique requires that the clinician ask the mother [caregiver] to: get down on the floor with her infant; follow her infant's lead; respond to her child, but only at the infant's initiative; not take over or direct the activity in any way; simply "watch, wait, and wonder.

The original instructions direct providers to spend 30 minutes on WWW and the rest of the time processing the caregiver's expectations. I tend to interject some conversation and exploration of the caregiver's observations throughout the whole session without setting aside specific time for processing. It is essential for interventions to feel natural to the provider. It will feel odd at first whenever we do something different, but as we move through it, we find a rhythm and make it our own.

Depending on the circumstance, we can play at the child's or caregiver's levels. When caregivers can and want to sit on the floor, we can sit with them and bring the play to the child's level. Other times, for accessibility or preference, we might raise the space to the caregiver's level (e.g., playing at a table instead of on the floor). This consideration is vital for caregivers who might not be able to get on the ground. As the therapist, I try to sit somewhat away from the dyad, allowing them space to be close to each other.

I introduced WWW to Yurisbel during one of our individual sessions before practicing it with Caleb present. She was concerned about his safety as he explored the room independently. We explored the concepts of safety and danger and identified situations where she would intervene. Sessions took place in a therapeutic playroom at my office.

Therapist: All right, how are you feeling about some watch, wait, and wonder?
Yurisbel: I think I'm ready for it.
Therapist: Great. As a reminder, we will spend some time just observing his play. Try to follow his lead as much as you can without questions or suggestions. I'll be right here with both of you.
Yurisbel: Bebe, you wanna play?
[Caleb was sitting on her lap. We waited several minutes, and he seemed curious but not ready to move.]
Yurisbel: What do I do? Should I move him so he can play?
Therapist: We can wait a bit more and see if he feels a little more comfortable. I wonder what would happen if you grabbed one of the toys and played alone but still close to him.
[Yurisbel grabs a truck and begins rolling it back and forth, making engine sounds.

Caleb looks interested in what his mom is doing. He moves from her lap to the floor beside her and says, "Truck." Yurisbel hands him the truck, and he carries it around the room. He starts grabbing toys and bringing them to his mom, and she asks, "What is this?" and "What color is it?"]
Yurisbel: I'm not supposed to ask questions, huh?
Therapist: It's a different way of being with him. Sometimes, I think about it as having play time versus having teaching time.
Yurisbel: Okay, play time then.
Caleb: Play.

We processed Yurisbel's feelings of anxiety at not giving directions throughout our time. She shared remembering her mother making her draw circles and lines when she was very young and thinking that she wanted to do this with Caleb. She needed to bridge some of her early experiences to her parenting while also seeing Caleb as a developing individual. I wondered whether some of the behaviors I was reading as intrusive were ways for her to keep her mother alive. In teaching, asking questions, and directing, she was trying to bring what she remembered about her mother. Using WWW provided a pathway to explore the ghosts and angels in the nursery. The angels represent experiences, whether in our awareness or outside, that are aspects of strengths gathered from our upbringing (Lieberman et al., 2005). As she made connections to her upbringing, she created space for Caleb's need to develop a sense of self and individuality.

INTERNAL RELATIONS

Our experiences and past relationships impact our ability to tune into ourselves and others (Frankland, 2010). Object relations theory (ORT) can help us understand how an individual develops reflective capacity. The theory holds that we internalize representations of our early caregivers that affect our relationships with others. What we experience, we tend to internalize and then re-enact. Chapter 2 explores ORT and its importance in caregiver–child relationships and well-being. A newborn is fully reliant on a caregiver. They have no understanding of emotions or the ability to meet their needs. When any discomfort happens, babies use crying as a way to signal that they need help. Newborns experience themselves as being part of the caregiver. This connected experience is not metaphorical. To the young baby, the caregiver is like the breath giving life. Closeness and comfort are basic emotional needs. Babies do not see themselves as separate from their caregivers until around six to nine months. Around this time, we might see some babies intentionally seeking to be closer to the caregiver and some separation anxiety marking the beginning of the recognition and fear that the caregiver might go away. As an internal sense of self begins to rise, the baby remains connected to their caregivers to make sense of the world and their emotional experience (Katrios, 2006). The caregiver is the reflector and the container of the child's experience.

Yurisbel was raised by her mother and grandmother. She reported that her mother was a political prisoner for a couple of years when she was a baby. Yurisbel described her grandmother as cold and distant. She reported that on one occasion she hurt her leg and could not walk. She brought it up with her grandmother, who responded, *"Serves you right, it's too bad it wasn't your head."* She continues, *"I just started to feel numb. Nothing bothered me after that. Lately, I feel like I lost control of my mind. I am angry and cry at everything."* In another session, Yurisbel reflected on how the loss of her mother impacted her ability to attune to her internal world.

Yurisbel: I want the anxiety and constant worry to go away.
Therapist: They are emotions hard to tolerate.
Yurisbel: I used to be able to before. This is not who I am. I was the one everyone looked up to when things got tough.

Therapist: Sometimes, our mind numbs a part of us so we can survive and do what needs to be done.

Yurisbel: It was like being numb to everything. No matter what happens.

Therapist: And a lot happened in your life. Many losses and little support. Feeling it might have been too much.

Yurisbel: I remember thinking about my mom when I was young and saying to myself, it's okay. I've got my aunt.

Therapist: Your mind knew what it needed to do and say to protect you.

Yurisbel: I want it to do it now. To protect me.

Therapist: The strategies our mind used when we were younger tend to not work as much as our life and situation shifts. There was no escape when you were young, so your mind found a way to help you avoid some of the pain.

Yurisbel: I just want to be good for Caleb. I want him to have a happy life.

Therapist: I can see how much you love him. Bringing a child into our lives can disrupt our internal world.

Yurisbel: I don't want to blame him.

Therapist: It's not his fault, and it's not yours either. With great love comes the fear of loss, and you've had a lifetime of it.

Yurisbel: Losing my mother. There has to be more feelings in there than numbness. I am scared to face it.

Therapist: We can take it step by step.

The dissociation from feelings was Yurisbel's mind's protection. She learned that she could not be disappointed if she did not feel pain or love. Her relationship with herself was disconnected. Adopting her son stirred up love and the fear of loss. Her mind could not protect her by separating her from the desire of wanting to raise Caleb. The desire to love her son was stronger. Our work entailed creating the capacity for her to grieve the parts of her that did not get to experience love, trust, and sensitivity. Through conversations, curiosity, and interpretations, she learned to trust that spectrums of fear and love can cohabit in the caregiver–child relationship.

Humans are reliant on each other for survival. We seek connection. The need for relationships looks different across people or cultures. What may be connecting to me might be disrespectful to you. Hence, the importance of curiosity in everything that we do. How we internalize representations of our caregivers also differs. Through an anti-oppressive lens, I can understand the client through their story and understanding of it.

JANEIL AND JALISSA'S STORY

Janeil is a 23-year-old mother to 8-month-old Jalissa. When Jalissa was 6 months old, she became involved with child protective services following a visit to the hospital after her father attacked her mom, Janiel. The hospital became concerned for Jalissa, as she was present during the attack and presented inconsolable. The dyad was residing in a shelter following a break from the relationship with Jalissa's father. Janeil was referred by the court system to participate in parenting classes, and no other services were recommended. The shelter referred Janeil to counseling following concerns of depression.

Janeil is a Black woman raised in the foster care system. She reported being permanently removed from her family's care when she was 7. When she was 3, Janeil's mother left her with a neighbor for a few days. Janeil reported that this was her first involvement with CPS, as her mother abandoned her. She was removed at age 7 following verified sexual abuse and parental cocaine use. Janeil reported being sexually abused by multiple individuals, including family members and neighbors. Janeil obtained transitional housing when she aged out of the foster care system at 18. When she was 20, she met Jalissa's father, Omar. The relationship with Omar seemed optimistic, and Janeil decided to move in with him once her time at the transitional housing ended. The relationship became increasingly aggressive from the moment she moved in after six months of dating. Janeil reported that Omar's aggression escalated to physical violence during pregnancy. Intimate partner violence (IPV) worsens during pregnancy (American Academy of Obstetrics and Gynecology, 2012), and for many birthing people it begins during pregnancy. Janiel and her daughter moved into the current shelter following discharge from the hospital.

I held my first visit with Janeil in her room at the shelter. Finding a private space that would work was difficult. We arranged to meet when her roommate was out. Janeil still had some visible bruising from the attack. Janeil described feeling numb more often than not, having trouble getting out of bed, losing weight, and having nightmares. My job required me to give her a diagnosis to provide services. She met the criteria for Major Depressive Disorder with peripartum onset and for Posttraumatic Stress Disorder, Chronic. Janeil reported that she participated in counseling while in foster care and did not find it helpful. She reported having to take medications that changed how she felt and told me she would not retake meds.

Exploring Reflective Functioning

Janeil was carrying a lifetime of pain and disappointment. I felt hopeful that she was open to meeting with me, as she shared that many providers have failed her throughout her history. I was worried about Jalissa and her exposure to violence. I wondered how the baby was adjusting to all the scary changes that happened in a short amount of time. Having been exposed to IPV as a child, I needed to ensure that I could contain their story. We were also working cross-culturally, and I needed to create space for bringing social location into a situation where the client did not choose to work with me. Janiel seemed open to sharing and working together, but depression was a big concern, as it impacted her daily functioning. She explained having experienced depression most of her life but that the symptoms had significantly increased since the baby was born. Janiel was open to thinking about her feelings and history. She wondered whether she was depressed or stressed due to everything she had been through. She met Jalissa's needs for eating, changing, and sleeping but did not seem able to provide a stimulating environment for her.

Jalissa was calm, quiet, and lying in her car seat for most of the initial sessions. Her development across domains seemed at risk. Janiel reported that the pediatrician did not raise concerns about the baby's functioning. She reported being glad that the baby was quiet, as this allowed her time to rest and sleep. Eight-month-olds are generally active and on the move. I began to formulate a hypothesis about Janiel's CRF and her knowledge of age-appropriate expectations. I worried whether I could meet their needs. Janiel was referred to me for individual counseling, but her baby needed to be part of our work. After several sessions collecting information, I shared some of my concerns about Jalissa's development. Janiel reported that she did not want anyone else involved in Jalissa's care. Her experiences with the medical staff and CPS left a healthy distrust of others.

Moving into Intervention

I proposed a relational model of individual sessions intermixed with dyadic sessions to support Janiel, Jalissa, and their relationship. We explored how we would know if we needed more support than what I could provide. Some of our identified red flags were worsening depression, missing a lot of appointments, and the baby not advancing on her milestones. We worked together for 13 months, which included her transition out of the shelter system and into a permanent housing program.

The following is an excerpt from the beginning section of our work together.

Janiel: I've been trying to get out of the room more with the baby. She likes seeing other people. When they talk to her, she looks at them and smiles [appears sad].

Therapist: Hmm, I'm noticing some sadness behind that.

Janiel: She doesn't smile at me. Sometimes I try to talk to her, and she just stares or looks away.

Therapist: I see where the sadness comes from.

Janiel: I don't think I was born for this. Everyone here is excited to see her, and I am just tired.

Therapist: You are naming something depression tends to do. It drains our energy and makes it hard to do life.

Janiel: It's always been here, though. This feeling.

Therapist: It's not a new feeling. The things we are used to dealing with get so much harder when a baby joins our life.

Janiel: I see that now. I was doing so many things, and everything just fell apart. Life slowed down, but it kept going at the same time.

Therapist: You and your baby have had to survive a lot.

Janiel: I've been trying to think more about how I am feeling. I still think about everything all the time. Getting out of foster care, Omar, the baby, and the trip to the hospital. I get paralyzed when I think about it. It's like I go on autopilot.

As Janiel makes sense of her story, she is beginning to see trauma's impact on her well-being. I began to see her show interest in interacting with the baby, which was shadowed by feelings of rejection in interpreting that the baby liked others more than her. There was so much sadness as she shared that the baby smiled at others. I wondered if she was seeing in Jalissa the rejection she had experienced from her parents and caregivers during her time in the system. Had Janiel internalized a sense of badness and not being wanted? How did the relationship with Omar contribute to her sense of self and her relationship with the baby? I wanted to explore this with her to ensure we were collaborating in our work.

Therapist: We've spent some time talking about really painful experiences during the past sessions. How has it been for you to think about your life here with me?

Janiel: It's not fun. I didn't want to think about the past. I felt pretty numb when we started, and then I felt sad and angry about everything. Sometimes, I don't know what's the point.

Therapist: There's a lot to be sad and angry about.

Janiel: But what's the point? It'll never change. I'm not destined to have a good life [tearfully].

[Therapist leans in, takes a deep breath]

Janiel: I don't want to hope or get excited about what's next. I worry about my baby and what will happen to her. My life wasn't good. What if her life is also bad because of me? Everything I touch gets ruined.

Therapist: You've had to carry a lot of pain and disappointment.

Janiel: I don't want to carry it anymore.

The start of this conversation helped me understand her internal world a little better. Validating her experience was the beginning of deepening our work. Abuse can leave us with a destructive narrative about ourselves and the world. All her experiences of rejection helped build a destructive internal object. This

153

object was part of herself, always ready to tell her that she was not good enough. We learn to listen to the damaging voice out of a need for survival. In a dangerous upbringing, it is unsafe to hope. Hope leaves us disappointed. Survival also pushes the child who is being abused to internalize a sense of badness. This destructive internal object was the reality for Janiel. Depression also represented a lack of hope. If she stays in bed, she does not risk living life and being disappointed by others. As I began to formulate this hypothesis, I also needed to keep in mind and create space for the systemic barriers she had navigated throughout her life, like racism, growing up in foster care, and poverty. Many barriers will continue to be a part of her experience in the world long after we stop working together.

Holding Jalissa in Mind

The dyadic sessions shifted to multiple locations during our time together, depending on our access to privacy. We could set up on the bedroom floor when Janiel's roommate was not there. Other times, we found places to sit outside. Janiel was experiencing significant mental health needs, impacting her capacity to fully present for herself and her daughter. I wanted to give space for individual sessions while also supporting her daughter. I worried about their limited interactions. During some of our first dyadic sessions, Jalissa remained in the car seat and made minimal bids for her mother's attention. I needed to understand more about their dynamic.

Therapist: What kinds of things do you enjoy doing together?
Janiel: Watching TV, and she likes to eat.
Therapist: TV and eating sound like a good time.
Janiel: I think she pays attention to the show and always looks around when she hears the sound of food.
Therapist: Good ears there. I would love to hear more about her eating.
Janiel: She still does the bottle, but I gotta give her a little of what I am eating, or she gets mad. Even if she doesn't like it.
Therapist: She knows what she wants. She wants some of what Mommy likes, too.
Janiel: She likes sitting in her high chair to eat like a big girl.
Therapist: Oh goodness! How does she let you know?
Janiel: She'll point at it and make sounds like, "I'm ready for some food."
Therapist: I see you know what she likes. She's communicating, and you are listening.
Janiel: Yeah? I guess she is communicating, even with no words.
Therapist: They get pretty creative, letting us know what they want.
Janiel: [turns to Jalissa] I guess you're smart, huh?
Therapist: [speaking for the baby] I am mommy and you get me. I like that.

154

Part of my clinical motto is that any interaction between a caregiver and their baby is an opportunity for me to seek connection and pull at strengths. We want babies and caregivers to have face-to-face interactions that do not involve a screen. We know the research on screen time suggests less of it for little ones (Lammers et al., 2022). However, when the screen is how they spend time together, we need to see it for what it is: Their moment of connection. Janiel's story allowed me to sit with the idea of best practices versus what is best for this family at this moment. If caregivers are the experts in their children, I must step back, listen, and understand the meaning of their interactions. I know this is basic stuff for many of us, but how was it for you to see that her response to my initial question on their bonding was "TV?" I can say that for me my first response was judgment. I had to bring calm to my need to jump in and educate. Screen time remained our go-to bonding for many of our dyadic sessions.

The above excerpt also shows an example of the *speaking for the baby* intervention. The intervention is a way to bring the baby's thoughts and feelings into the room. It also promotes communication between babies and caregivers (Carter et al., 1991). Parental depression and PTSD can lead to lower vocalizations and overall communication between caregivers and children (Erickson et al., 2019). Untreated mental health conditions in the caregiver can impact the baby's development. We see some impact on Jalissa's development and some growth as Janiel begins holding her in mind. This is one of my favorite interventions because it is a less intrusive way of giving feedback in sessions. It brings the baby's internal world to the forefront. As with anything we try in counseling, we want to explore the appropriateness of the tool for the specific client. If you notice a reaction to using speaking for the baby, explore the meaning with the client. You can say, *"I noticed when I talked as if the baby, you had a reaction. This kind of talk is one I use sometimes in counseling, and I want to ensure this is a collaborative space. How was that for you?"* There is so much that we do not know. It will be impossible to predict the goodness of fit of a particular intervention for everyone. This reality brings us back to the importance of reflection and tracking moment-to-moment shifts in the session.

In this example, I used speaking for the baby to bring connection and support back and forth in communication for the dyad. Reciprocity is vital to building nurturing relationships (Erickson et al., 2019). When a baby sends a signal, the caregiver reads the cue and sends a signal back. The dyad enters a dance that can become a game or meet another developmental need. It is one of the earliest forms of active communication for little ones. Reciprocity requires CRF. The caregiver must see their baby as a being with desires and wishes that must be communicated and understood. Understanding the child's unique characteristics helps increase motivation for getting to know them, strengthening the relationship (Zero to Three, 2016). A reciprocal and rewarding relationship supports the child and the caregiver's mental health. Caregiving young children is difficult. When fun and joy are low, it becomes harder to endure the challenging moments.

A Few Sessions Later

Janiel: Do you know when she's going to talk?

Therapist: That's a great question. It's a little different for every baby. Many say their very first word at around a year. How do you think she's doing?

Janiel: She makes lots of sounds and has been screaming loudly.

Therapist: Oh yeah! Loud screaming and even screeching are common. She's learning to use her voice.

Janiel: That's what that is?

Therapist: Yeah, she makes sounds and gets to learn about her environment and how to get some connection with others.

Janiel: She has been doing it and looks at me. I think she was laughing at me the other day.

Therapist: It does feel good when mommy looks at you. Why do you think she was laughing?

Janiel: I fell asleep, and she woke me up.

Therapist: That's a good example of her learning about the world. Loud noises wake people up.

Janiel: I guess that's good.

Therapist: I wonder what you thought the loud noises meant.

Janiel: I thought something was wrong with her.

Therapist: You were worried. I'm glad you shared it with me. This is also a space to talk about any concerns, questions, or worries you have.

Janiel: I think I took a long time to talk. Maybe it'll be the same for her.

Therapist: Maybe. Every baby moves at their own beat. Would it be helpful to think about some things you can do together to support her communication?

Janiel: Yeah. What kind of things?

Therapist: Little things that can also be fun. Before discussing some options, I would love to learn what you already do together for communication.

Janiel: Well, we've been going outside, so she hears other people. She also hears the TV and pays attention.

Therapist: Those are definitely strategies we can build upon. Making sure that she is hearing words.

Janiel: So, it's not so bad then. She hears plenty of that.

Therapist: It might be good to also add other options like reading, singing, and talking to her.

Janiel: It's weird to talk to her. She pays attention, but I don't know if she understands.

Therapist: She probably understands more than we think. It can feel awkward at first to talk to a baby. Some people find it helpful to just narrate your actions or name things around you.

Janiel: [turns to baby] We're in therapy. It's really hot out here.

Therapist: Look at her looking at you. She likes your voice. I have a little fan we use if you want to take her out of the car seat.

[Janiel takes the baby out of the car seat and sits her in front of her. Jalissa begins kicking and moving her arms.]

Therapist: Ahhh! Feels good to be outside.

Janiel: She is moving around so much more.

Therapist: Talking about moving, does she like music?

Janiel: Oh, she loves it. She will kick around and dance.

Therapist: Music and singing are great tools for communication. What kind of music do you both like?

Janiel: She likes it all. She's a fan of mommy's music and *Baby Shark*.

Therapist: We can listen to some music together if you'd like.

We spent the rest of the session searching for songs and seeing how Jalissa reacted to the music. In this case, the screen became a tool for deeper connection. Janiel's concern about the baby's communication was our port of entry to strengthening the relationship. The more Janiel became interested in Jalissa, the more she started catching up on her milestones. There was joy and fear for Janiel as she learned about what her baby's behaviors meant. She was beginning to feel excitement for their interaction while worrying about things that could go wrong. By this time we had been working together for almost two months, and Jalissa was still spending time in the car seat during our sessions. You can see in the above excerpt that I directly offered an opportunity for Janiel to take Jalissa out of the car seat. I wondered whether Janiel needed a sense of permission to interact with the baby. Janiel was unsure how to play or talk with her daughter and needed guidance on trusting herself. I later learned that Janiel spent several years in a group home that included babies. She told me how the babies spent the day in bouncers or car seats. I learned that keeping Jalissa in her car seat was what she thought made sense. We needed time for her to explore options and to see what would work for her and her baby.

SUMMARY

Reflective capacity helps caregivers bridge to their child's world and respond in sensitive and attuned ways. When caregivers can hold their child in mind, relationships can deepen. Watch, wait, and wonder, and speaking for the baby are strategies therapists can use to support reflective capacity. In Yurisbel's story, we see how the ghosts from her past present in her relationship with Caleb. Gentle exploration of past history and the therapist's own reflective capacity are vital to exploring object relations. In Janiel and Jalissa's story, we see the ghosts of past trauma and their influence on her capacity to hold hope about her future. When therapists can partner with clients and their strengths, positive change can happen.

REFERENCES

American Academy of Obstetrics and Gynecology. (2012). Intimate partner violence. https://www.acog.org/clinical/clinical-guidance/committee-opinion/articles/2012/02/intimate-partner-violence

Carter, S. L., Osofsky, J. D., & Hann, D. M. (1991). Speaking for the baby: A therapeutic intervention with adolescent mothers and their infants. *Infant Mental Health Journal*, *12*(4), 291–301. https://doi.org/10.1002/1097-0355(199124)12:4<291::AID-IMHJ2280120403>3.0.CO;2-3

Cohen, N. J., Muir, E., Lojkasek, M., Muir, R., Parker, J. C., Barwick, M., & Brown, M. (1999). Watch, wait, and wonder: Testing the effectiveness of a new approach to mother–infant psychotherapy. *Infant Mental Health Journal*, *20*(4), 429–451. https://doi.org/10.1002/(SICI)1097-0355(199924)20:4<429::AID-IMHJ5>3.0.CO;2-Q

Erickson, N., Julian, M., & Muzik, M. (2019). Perinatal depression, PTSD, and trauma: Impact on mother–infant attachment and interventions to mitigate the transmission of risk. *International Review of Psychiatry*, *31*(3), 245–263. https://doi.org/10.1080/09540261.2018.1563529

Fraiberg, S., Adelson, E., & Shapiro, V. (1975). Ghosts in the nursery: A psychoanalytic approach to the problems of impaired infant–mother relationships. *Journal of the American Academy of Child Psychiatry 14*(3). 387–421. https://doi.org/10.1016/s0002-7138(09)61442-4

Frankland, A. G. (2010). *The little psychotherapy book: Object relations in practice.* Oxford University Press.

Heffron, M. C., & Murch, T. (2010) *Reflective supervision and leadership in infant and early childhood programs.* Zero to Three.

Katrios, T. (2006). The object as an agent of mentalization. *Journal of Theory and Criticism*, *14*, 71–82. https://doi.org/10.26262/gramma.v14i0.6514

Lammers, S. M., Woods, R. J., Brotherson, S. E., Deal, J. E., & Platt, C. A. (2022). Explaining adherence to American academy of pediatrics screen time recommendations with caregiver awareness and parental motivation factors: Mixed methods study. *Journal of Medical and Internet Research Pediatrics and Parenting*, *5*(2), e29102. https://doi.org/10.2196/29102

Lieberman, A. F., Padrón, E., Van Horn, P., & Harris, W. M. (2005). Angels in the nursery: The intergenerational transmission of benevolent parental influences. *Infant Mental Health Journal*, *26*(6), 504–520. https://doi.org/10.1002/imhj.20071

Luyten, P., Nijssens, L., Fonagy, P., & Mayes, L. C. (2017). Parental reflective functioning: Theory, research, and clinical applications. *The Psychoanalytic Study of the Child*, *70*(1), 174–199. https://doi.org/10.1080/00797308.2016.1277901

Madsen, E. B., Væver, M. S., Egmose, I., Krong, M. T., Haase, T. W., de Moor, M. H. M., & Karstoft, K. (2023). Parental reflective functioning in first-time parents and associations with infant socioemotional development. *Journal of Child and Family Studies*. https://doi.org/10.1007/s10826-023-02565-5

Mental Health America. (n.d.). Position statement 49: Perinatal mental health. https://mhanational.org/issues/position-statement-49-perinatal-mental-health

Muir, E. (1992). Watching, waiting, and wondering: Applying psychoanalytic principles to mother–infant intervention. *Infant Mental Health Journal*, *13*(4), 319–328. https://doi.org/10.1002/1097-0355(199224)13:4<319::AID-IMHJ 2280130407>3.0.CO;2-2

Postpartum Support International. (n.d.). Adoptive and birth mothers. https://tinyurl.com/yhd99vkm

Slade, A. (2005). Parental reflective functioning: An introduction. *Journal of Attachment and Human Development*, *7*(3), 269–281. https://doi.org/10.1080/14616730500245906

Stroud, B., & Morgan, M. M. (2014). Basics of counseling in infant–parent and early childhood mental health. In K. Brandt, B. Perry, S. Seligman, & E. Tronick (Eds.), *Infant and early childhood mental health: Core concepts and clinical practice*. American Psychiatric Association.

Tenets Initiative. (2018). Diversity-informed tenets for work with infants, children & families/Principios informados en la diversidad para trabajar con bebés, niños, niñas y familias. Irving Harris Foundation. https://diversityinformedtenets.org/download-the-tenets/

Zero to Three. (2016). *DC:0–5™: Diagnostic classification of mental health and developmental disorders of infancy and early childhood*. Author.

CHAPTER TEN

Play as a Pathway to Healing

Babies seek connection from the moment they are born. They turn their heads towards voices they heard frequently while in the womb soon after delivery (Lee & Kisilevsky, 2014). With time, babies begin reaching and smiling as a way to seek fun interaction with others. Children are hard-wired for the dance of playful communication with those around them. Play is how little ones sense their environment and connect to their world (Landreth, 2012). Although many of us are born with this innate drive for play, we tend to lose it as we grow up. Play requires a capacity to be in the moment. Colonization and capitalism chip away at our ability to connect with ourselves and others. Dominant culture permeates our childhoods, pushing us to focus, learn, and find ways to make money (e.g., survive). The barriers imposed by our capitalistic society make it impossible for us to value rest, entertainment, and fun highly. When individuals transition into caregiverhood, they often find that play no longer comes easily, nor does it create the joy it brings to their children. Reconnecting with playful delight is vital to nurturing, loving, and healthy relationships. Therapists looking to integrate a relational model into their work must find ways to support play as a pathway to healing and communication between caregiver and child. This chapter explores tools for bringing therapeutic play to caregivers and their little ones in and outside the counseling space.

PLAY THERAPY

Providers working from a relational and anti-oppressive approach have many competing treatment focuses. We want to honor the caregiver's interest and meet their individual needs. We must also find ways to bring the child's interests

DOI: 10.4324/9781003286394-14

and needs to the forefront. This second piece is one that often gets forgotten in perinatal treatment. As perinatal therapists, we support the caregiver's well-being and might fail to keep the child in mind. When working with caregivers, our capacity to think relationally must be present in all treatment modalities. Children need to be seen and heard to thrive. Holding the child in mind is especially important when children cannot communicate their needs or understand their world. Babies and young children rely on the adults around them to help them make sense. The emotional health of caregivers and children is intrinsically connected. When caregivers are not well, babies suffer, and vice versa. Integrating play into the relationships between caregivers, babies, and toddlers yields profound developmental and relational benefits. It is also an anti-oppressive way to reduce barriers by having one provider support the caregiver–child dyad. This kind of intentional play goes beyond mere entertainment. It is a form of *being with* that offers emotional bonding and supports cognitive growth and the development of essential life skills. Development takes place throughout the lifespan. Emotional bonding is not only a task for babies but also one for caregivers.

Play therapy helps children express themselves, communicate their emotions, and work through psychological challenges through play, the agent of change (Association for Play Therapy, n.d.). A child-directed play model allows the baby to lead the interaction by considering their emotional and developmental needs (Guerney, 2001). It provides a tool for caregivers to understand their child's world by observing and following the lead in their communication. A common myth about early childhood is that pre-verbal children do not have much to say. When we add the layer of systemic barriers, depression, birth trauma, or other mental health complications, it can feel impossible for some caregivers to bridge authentic connections without appropriate support. Part of our goal in introducing play is to enhance reciprocity within the relationship. Reciprocity refers to back-and-forth attuned interactions between the caregiver and child (Harvard Center on the Developing Child, n.d.). Reciprocal interactions are the key to supporting development and building relationships.

Julian, a 15-month-old bi-racial child, looks at his father and says, "Ball." His father looks back, smiles, and repeats the word. Julian then points to the ball and smiles as his father points back to it. His father asks, "Do you want the ball?" Julian smiles brightly and reaches for the ball. Reciprocity can only happen if two people are on the same page. As Julian bids for his father's attention, we can see how they enter a brief dance of communication. Julian is asking for more than the ball. He is asking for engagement. How does a caregiver know if they are on the same page as their baby, toddler, or preschooler? As discussed in Chapter 9, reflective practice is the road to connection. The caregiver's capacity to think, "*What does my child want and need*?" is the compass to the therapeutic benefits of play.

We can support the caregiver's reflective capacity by talking and exploring the metaphorical or underlying meaning of how children play. A 9-year-old who experienced a significant trauma might find themselves re-enacting different aspects of the trauma through the toys they use and the themes presented. Play therapy with very young children will look different from older ones who can create stories. For babies and young children, play with their caregivers will include singing, reading stories, cuddles, and other loving touch-based activities. We engage when the child is ready, and we stop when we attune to their cues of disinterest. In her book *Infant play therapy*, Courtney (2020) stated that "Infant play therapies are informed by the fields of neuroscience and infant mental health, are culturally sensitive, and utilize the therapeutic powers of play to effect positive change for the infant and parental (or caregiver) relational system and social environment" (p. 7). In my journey of becoming and being a play therapist, I witnessed the magic of the therapeutic powers of play on my life and the lives of children and families. The therapeutic powers of play refer to how play itself is the facilitator of change (Drewes & Schaefer, 2016). The playful dynamic between the caregiver and their child is the therapeutic factor that we want to support.

Something I heard in many of my play therapy trainings was that caregivers are their children's best toys. This idea goes back to the importance of the relationship. At the same time, much of the focus of play therapy is on supporting the child's needs. I invite us to think about play therapy as a way to support the caregiver, the child, and their relationship. All three pieces (or more if we involve other individuals and relationships) are vital for the therapist to consider. A caregiver's capacity to connect with their child significantly protects the mental health of all involved (Luyten et al., 2017). Mutual delight is vital for healthy relationships. Good enough joy, nurturing, and fun provide the cushion for difficult moments where stress increases, requiring caregivers to provide co-regulation.

REFLECTING ON OUR EXPERIENCES

Before we explore tools and ways to bring play into the caregiver–child space, let us examine our relationship with play and playfulness. This practice is a way to continuously hold in mind Tenet 1, self-awareness (Tenets Initiative, 2018). Please take some time to reflect, write, or draw upon these questions:

- What is your level of comfort with play and playfulness in your life? What about your work?

_____

_____

_____

- What do you remember about playing as a child?

  _____

  _____

  _____

- What types of games did you enjoy growing up?

  _____

  _____

  _____

- Who played with you?

  _____

  _____

  _____

- When and how did playing stop in your life?

  _____

  _____

  _____

- How do you connect with play as an adult?

  _____

  _____

  _____

- If you are not a play or a child therapist, what comes up as you think about introducing play in your work?

  _____

  _____

  _____

- If you are a play or a child therapist, how do you engage caregivers in therapeutic play?

  _____

  _____

  _____

PATHWAY TO HEALING AND COMMUNICATION

Play is a natural means of communication for children. It creates an environment where they can learn to make sense of the world. Play enables serve-and-return interaction, which becomes the basis for communication. Play is what helps the dyad. It is the medicine. While play may facilitate a discussion with a caregiver, this is not our aim. The goal is to be in the present moment with the family. Play is a way to embody several of the Diversity Informed Tenets (See Chapter 1 for a complete list). Our capacity as providers to support therapeutic play contributes to a welcoming, protective, and nurturing environment, as described in the Tenet, "Champion children's rights globally" (Tenets Initiative, 2018, para. 2). If *play is children's language and toys are their words*, then play helps us uphold Tenet 7, "Support families in their preferred language" (para. 7). Although Tenet 7 refers to using the family's native language, babies and young children are family members and need connection in a language that makes sense for them. Providers supporting adult populations can use play therapy tools to connect with children at their developmental level.

Effective communication is essential for the caregiver–child relationship. It is particularly crucial during the early developmental stages when babies fully rely on caregivers to make sense of the world. Play therapy provides a medium for caregivers to observe and interpret non-verbal cues, fostering a deeper understanding of their child's emotions and needs. A gesture like pointing or turning their heads when their loved one walks by becomes the ground for exploration. When a child points at something and the caregiver looks and points back, the baby experiences being seen and heard. The back and forth between caregiver and child forms the basis for healthy social and emotional development, laying the groundwork for future relationships and emotional regulation (Nijssens et al., 2018). These playful interactions offer a safe space for babies and young children to express themselves, even before they can articulate their feelings through words. As babies express themselves, caregivers can learn about their baby's personality, needs, and desires.

Through play, caregivers learn to be sensitive to their child's cues, adapt to their preferences, and engage in reciprocal interactions, promoting healthy communication patterns (Harvard Center on the Developing Child, n.d.; Yogman et al., 2018). As caregivers respond to their child's signals during play, they strengthen the child's sense of agency and a belief that their needs matter. For connection to happen, people need to be on the same page. Attuned, playful interactions establish a secure emotional foundation where trust, comfort, and safety are cultivated. These interactions are responsive, sensitive, and reliable more often than not. Babies learn that their world is predictable.

The benefits are not for the baby alone. The caregiver also experiences the gift of this connection as they understand their child and their vital role in each other's lives. When there is joy and pleasure in a relationship, well-being improves. These interactions can foster security for the caregiver and baby, leading to increased confidence, reduced anxiety, and the development of a robust internal working model for future relationships among all family members.

The reality of the caregiver's role in a child's life can place immense pressure on caregivers. Sensitivity and a capacity to bond do not come naturally for many caregivers. Mental health complications impact our ability to be present, regulate our emotions, and feel connected to others (Nijssens et al., 2018). Even when there is no mental health complication, caregivers are meeting and getting to know their children at each stage of development. As providers, we need to ensure that we are attuning to the readiness of the caregiver to hear and apply different forms of play. When people feel at their worst, the thought of having one more thing to do can be unbearable. We need to introduce play in a way that the caregiver can digest. Providing too much too soon can be overwhelming. A gentle introduction to play can support the caregiver's sense of competency.

In some cases, for the caregiver to demonstrate sensitivity, they might have to experience it from us as providers. This idea links us back to the parallel process (See Chapter 5) and *how we are* when we support caregivers. Here are two questions for us providers to consistently explore:

- Are we attuned to the caregiver's needs and holding them in mind as we encourage them to think about their children?
- How do I know when I need to slow down with this family?

CAREGIVER'S LEVEL OF COMFORT WITH PLAY

Our level of comfort with play can depend on many factors. You had an opportunity earlier to reflect on your relationship with play. What did you notice about yourself? What do you imagine can impact a caregiver's comfort?

I was not a natural at play as a starting therapist. I was uncomfortable during my training and felt self-conscious about being silly and seen by others. When I reflect on my experiences with play, I remember playing with toys and creating stories while living in Venezuela. I arrived in the U.S.A. at the age of 10 and was about to start the sixth grade. I realized my classmates did not play with dolls, blocks, or other toys. If they did, we certainly did not talk about it. As is true for many immigrant and refugee children, we did not bring our toys or other meaningful belongings from back home. I remember my first winter holiday in the U.S.A. I got a Bingo set as my only gift. I realized my time playing was done. I was "allowed" to play but not in an imaginative, story-filled way. On my second Christmas here, we got to bring bags of toys from a local church, which allowed us to have gifts that winter. My bag was filled with teddy bears, many of which I still have. Although I appreciated them, there was no more playing for me. They were decorations and maybe a way to remain connected with playfulness.

We all have a story about what play meant to us and how it stopped. U.S. dominant culture values excelling and productivity over rest and enjoyment. Capitalism tries to sell us the message of work now and play later. Connecting with our playful self requires bypassing the social conditioning of constantly minding how others see us. I am wondering if the experience of "not calling too much attention to yourself" is universal. Being too loud, rowdy, and visible is dangerous for Black and Brown children and those holding other identities, like living in poverty or a larger body. Many children of color stop playing as a mechanism for navigating systemic racism and other injustices (Rowland-Shea & Doshi, 2020; Scott, 2017). For those of us whose childhood involved being parentified or needing to survive trauma, play can feel unnatural and, in some cases, unsafe. It is not an easy feat for many of us. Letting go and being in the moment can feel and be scary. We may not be aware of our scared feelings and interpret them as a lack of interest. As providers, we may also inaccurately see a caregiver's sense of survival as a lack of interest in their child's feelings. What caregivers bring into their relationship with their children impacts interactions. As we understand the caregiver's relationship with play, our starting point is attunement to their history through an anti-oppressive lens. It can help us guide conversations and maintain cultural humility. Before providing psychoeducation or recommendations on different play strategies, we want to know:

- How is this for the caregiver?
- How does the caregiver understand the meaning and purpose of playful interactions?
- What were their early experiences with play?

RAMON AND JULIAN'S STORY

Ramon came to see me when his son Julian was 5 months old (the same child from the above story). Ramon reported feeling angry all the time, isolating from loved ones, and increasing the use of alcohol in the evening. He said he had been having intrusive thoughts and nightmares about his daughter Inaya, who died at birth eight years ago. Perinatal mental health complications in men are less studied and understood than in women and mothers (Scarff, 2019). There are no unified criteria for complications like postnatal depression in men, but we know it is common, impacting about one in ten fathers.

Similarly, men's experience of perinatal loss is often forgotten by research, providers, and even loved ones (Mota et al., 2023). Charles Robinson shares his experience of paternal perinatal loss in an interview with James Harris, founder of Men to Heal (Harris, 2020). In the interview, Robinson described how loved ones focused their attention on his partner, unintentionally contributing to the erasure of his experience. Societal discourses, like men do not get depressed and need to be strong for their partner, coupled with other systemic barriers, impact their capacity to seek, access, and receive treatment.

Ramon is a 33-year-old South American man who migrated to the U.S.A. with his parents when he was 12. He is married to Julian's mother, Valentina, and they are in a polyamorous relationship. Ramon explained that he is receiving support from his partners. When asked about his family of origin, he reported that although he is close to his family, they do not know he is polyamorous. He noted that one of his partners encouraged him to seek therapy following an episode where he began screaming and punched a wall. Valentina's partner, Lucia, is currently living in their home, supporting Julian's care.

During the assessment, Ramon reported that Julian was a surprise pregnancy, as they were told that Valentina could not become pregnant following Inaya's death. He said he was unconcerned about Julian's well-being, as *"He is very young."* One of the myths of infancy is that environment does not affect young children. This misconception can create a lot of unintentional harm to the child's developing brain and relationships. I shared with Ramon my interest in the whole family's well-being. As he was open to hearing more, I shared brief psychoeducation on young children, trauma, and socio-emotional development. Ramon was unsure about bringing Julian to counseling sessions. He was concerned about his family's judgment and did not want Julian to have a mental health history. I respected his lead and explored the possibility of keeping him in mind during our time. We discussed the impact of bringing Julian up in treatment while avoiding pathologizing him and upholding his concern about not giving his son his own chart or medical record. This idea might be tricky when enough concerns arise, suggesting a need for additional support, such as a referral to another provider, like an occupational therapist. I shared this concern with him, and we agreed to bring Julian up in session without him joining us yet.

I asked him to share about how Julian communicates and how their relationship has been doing. Ramon shared that Julian was not yet communicating much. He stated that the past month had been emotionally painful, as he thought about Inaya almost every time he looked at his son. The beginning of treatment focused on understanding how Inaya's loss impacted Ramon and his relationship with Julian. I also wondered about Ramon's understanding of child development and his interest in interacting with Julian. In one of our earlier sessions, I encouraged Ramon to spend some time observing Julian and how he plays. He returned to the session, sharing that the observation was uneventful, stating, *"he ate, slept, and cried."* When I asked about his involvement in responding to those needs, he shared that Valentina and Lucia have been Julian's main caregivers, as they were *"better with him."*

I wanted to find a way to encourage a nurturing relationship between Ramon and Julian without adding to feelings of inadequacy or creating harm to the family's ecosystem. Each time we met, I found ways to explore how he was holding Julian in mind. We spent sessions discussing early relational health and play with babies and its impact on caregiver mental health. After a few weeks, we revisited the idea of bringing Julian into our sessions.

Therapist: We've spent some time talking about bonding in your relationship with Julian. I wonder what it would be like to talk about revisiting Julian joining one of our sessions.

Ramon: I haven't driven alone with him yet.

Therapist: It's funny how we can drive so much, yet it can feel so different when our tiny baby is in the back.

Ramon: Seriously.

Therapist: If it feels good to you, I have a few options we can explore.

[Ramon nods]

Therapist: I have some ideas for activities we can do together. We can meet online, so you don't have to worry about bringing him to the office. We can also meet here, and Valentina can join us, so you don't drive with him alone.

Ramon: I like the online idea.

Therapist: Great. Both you and the baby can remain where you are most comfortable and where it can feel more natural to be together.

Ramon: What would we be doing?

Therapist: We can do some playful activities specific to babies. We can prepare and talk more about them before we meet with Julian. How are you feeling about this plan?

Ramon: It's not bad. I am willing to try anything that will help.

Therapist: And I am here to support you. I want to ensure that whatever we do feels comfortable and we collaborate on it. Before moving forward, can we talk a little more about the session structure and how you feel?

Ramon feels unsure about caring for Julian alone. Part of this feeling might be due to him taking a secondary role in caregiving at home. Another part sounded like anxiety, as he shared that he is not driving alone with the baby just yet. I wondered how the trauma of losing Inaya was intermixing his capacity to feel capable of protecting his child. By exploring his feelings and our collaboration, I wanted to support him as a present voice in our clinical relationship. Ramon mentioned that the first child he had held was Inaya. His experience caring for children was limited. Culturally, Ramon explored how men in his upbringing and community are not involved in childrearing. He reported that he often heard his mother saying that his father never changed a diaper. Ramon shared wanting to be an involved father. I introduced a directive play-based tool to give him something tangible to build upon. I chose FirstPlay® as our first intervention.

FirstPlay® is a play therapy model that uses loving touch and storytelling to enhance the parent–child relationship (Courtney, 2020). In this manualized model, providers teach parents a story and different massage movements to use with their babies. The provider demonstrates the massage movements on a doll while the caregiver massages the baby. As we go through the FirstPlay® movements, the therapist supports attunement, sensitivity, and responsiveness by giving verbal and non-verbal feedback to the caregiver. One beautiful aspect of this model is the provider's capacity to be flexible in allowing the baby to lead the interaction.

Partnering in Play

Ramon shared feelings of interest and hesitation. He reported that the baby sometimes cried while he carried him and felt that Julian preferred everyone else over him. He felt frustrated at not knowing how to care for his son. We explored the root of some of those feelings: culture, family of origin, depression, Inaya's loss, and the newness of this experience. Reflecting on what impacted his experience with his son before moving into play allowed Ramon to choose how our sessions proceeded. We had an opportunity to practice the story and the massage movements on dolls before Julian joined us. The preparation sessions helped us set the stage and to give the caregiver an understanding of what we are doing so that they can have a sense of competency in the process when the child is present. The preparation sessions before the baby joins can take as long as the caregivers need. Ramon and I took about five sessions to discuss concerns before "rehearsing" our play strategy.

Therapist: We have our dolls ready for FirstPlay®. How is this feeling for you?

Ramon: I feel kinda silly. I ain't even gonna lie.

Therapist: It is not every day that we sit with another adult to play with a doll. It is a stretch past our comfort zone.

Ramon: I don't think I've ever played with a doll.

Therapist: We don't tend to socialize boys to play with dolls in our culture.

Ramon: Oh, that's true. I was told, "usted es un hombrecito los hombrecitos juegan a camiones" (you're a little man, little men play with trucks).

Therapist: Much of our work as adults is reparenting ourselves and choosing what stories we want to continue with our children and which need to shift.

Ramon: I want him to play with everything.

Therapist: Yes. This is our way in. Modeling and providing him with loving experiences that are not only good for him but for you as well.

Ramon: No one prepares you for this.

Therapist: Mmm-hmm.

Ramon: I guess there is no manual, huh?

Therapist: No specific manual for each child. You have an internal compass that tells you when something feels good and doesn't. Babies do, too. You are figuring out what Julian's compass says.

Ramon: It's hard to know what he wants, since he can't talk.

Therapist: Yes, it makes us detectives looking for clues. This is what we do with this type of play. We have a flow, but really, we will move at Julian's pace.

We have to figure out what he is trying to communicate with his body, movements, and sounds.

Ramon: It's going to be way easier with the doll.

Therapist: The doll doesn't really have any needs. It can help us understand the movements and get the awkwardness of being silly out of the way.

We took time to review baby cues for readiness to play. I wanted to get a sense of how Ramon understood Julian's signals. He was able to name crying and pushing away as cues of disinterest. We reviewed the story in the FirstPlay® manual and practiced the massage movements on our dolls.

Therapist: Now that we went through it. How is this feeling?

Ramon: It was good to laugh. I hope he likes it.

Therapist: Laughter is good for the soul. He will let us know which parts he likes and which not. Sometimes, it is a matter of preference or getting comfortable with the massage movements.

Ramon: Can I practice with him this week?

Therapist: Of course! You are welcome to take the manual with the story or to create your own song, stories, or massage movements.

Ramon: What about the songs I like?

Therapist: Oooh! Please say more.

Ramon: I was thinking *La Vaca* [a well-known merengue song].

Therapist: That sounds like a lot of fun.

Ramon: I was playing it for him the other day, and he was dancing to it.

Therapist: Great, I love it. You know what he likes. This is what it's about, finding what makes sense for you and your little guy.

Our steps to slow down, practice, and check in allowed Ramon to explore what felt natural. The goal of any play-based activity in counseling is for it to make sense for the caregiver and the child. Both parties are equally crucial in conceptualizing fun, joy, and nurturing. Ramon and Julian joined the next session remotely. Julian was smiling, sitting on his father's lap. Ramon shared that he could play the song with Julian and did leg and arm movements. He reported that Valentina and Lucia were interested in learning FirstPlay®. I was excited about this idea and wanted to ensure that Ramon continued to feel competent in his caregiving and relationship with his son. We began setting up for our activity.

Therapist: Hi, Julian! I am so happy to meet you. You are very smiley.

Ramon: He's been smiling at everyone.

Therapist: You see him seeking those connections.

Ramon: Do you want to see what we've been doing?

Therapist: Yes.

Ramon: Okay. Let me look for the song.

Therapist: I can cue it up for us if you'd like so y'all can get ready.

Ramon: [talking to Julian] Baby, do you want to dance?

[Julian responded by kicking his legs and looking at his dad. When the music started, Ramon began by swinging Julian from side to side. Julian began giggling as his father made cow noises and a silly face. Ramon had also made up some fun leg movements for Julian, where he placed his hands in front of Julian's feet. Julian would then kick his father's hands. It was a lovely back-and-forth connection that created some belly laughs.]

Therapist: I can see how much you both enjoy each other.

Ramon: He just loves music.

Therapist: He does, and he loves being with you.

Ramon: I guess he does.

Therapist: How is it to see that?

Ramon: That he loves me? It feels good. Like I haven't messed him up.

Therapist: That critical voice tries to come through.

Ramon: I am trying not to let it. I see him smiling and just having a great time. I want that for him and me.

We spent the rest of the session playing with different songs, creating massage-like movements, and working on attunement. Julian told us when he needed a break in stimulation and one to eat. As the session ended, I wanted to revisit Ramon's comment on having others join our sessions.

Therapist: What would it be like for you if Valentina and Lucia were to join us?

Ramon: They have been worried about me, and I think they are trying to be supportive.

Therapist: It's nice to have people that care about us.

Ramon: Yeah, I am feeling better, but don't want to let my guard down.

Therapist: All relationships need a bit of tending, those we have with others and those we have with ourselves.

Ramon: I hadn't thought about how self-critical I was. Nothing I did felt right.

Therapist: Grief, sadness, and anxiety can do that.

Ramon: For real. I was thinking everyone was criticizing me when it was really me.

Therapist: How is that critical voice sounding when you think about Julian and being a father?

Ramon: It is okay when we are alone, but not so much when other people are looking at me.

Therapist: Hmmm, and we are talking about bringing some other sets of eyes into our space.

Ramon: Yeah, like they are going to know I am a fraud of a dad.

Therapist: That internal voice is really critical.

Ramon: What do I do?

Therapist: I think this is the doing. Talking about it. Being curious about where it is coming from when it rises. Continuing to parent yourself and your child.

Ramon: Forever huh?

Therapist: Yes and … It gets easier the more awareness and practice we put into it.

Ramon: I guess that's true. I feel less bad.

Therapist: Knowing that it probably will feel uncomfortable, how ready do you feel to invite someone else into our space?

Ramon: I want to. Maybe we can start with Valentina, one person instead of two.

Therapist: Great. We can plan what we will do together just like we did before we brought Julian into our space.

Ramon: I thought we would do the massage.

Therapist: Absolutely. We can also do something else if you want, like play with toys, sing, or use the bubbles machine. It can be up to you and Julian to decide.

We have many options for encouraging play. Ensuring our environment is conducive to babies and toddlers is a starting point. For providers meeting with clients in person, having toys, a changing table, and a place to dispose of diapers are ways to welcome little ones. Those of us meeting with clients online must be intentional about how we welcome babies into the space. You can choose to have some playful things in your background or be available to interact with the child when they come in. The best activity will be the one that both caregiver and child enjoy.

Reflection on Ramon and Julian's Story

Ramon and his relationship with Julian were struggling when counseling first started. Ramon carried a lot of pain from his past and the loss of Inaya into his relationship with his son. His internal critic was ever-alert, constantly questioning his capacity to care for Julian. Play was the facilitator in building a stronger relationship and sense of competence for Ramon. The more he saw that his son communicated and responded to him, the better he started feeling. I introduced an infant play therapy model, which Ramon made his own. The goal of any intervention we try with families is that it works for them, and that they can mold it to meet their needs.

The transition to parenthood is demanding. It is lonely when everything changes and we are not connecting with our children. It is a familiar road that many people find themselves navigating. As you support families, consider ways to bridge play and fun into each session. I want to invite the notion that play is accessible to all. It will sometimes look different from caregiver to caregiver, child to child, or provider to provider. The power of play therapy is transtheoretical (Drewes & Schaefer, 2016). We can move across different playful models and activities to effect change. Think about what is accessible to you at this moment. Can you attend an infant play therapy or an infant mental health training or program? If you can, then do that and consult with other providers serving this population. If right now is not the right time or you are not interested in being a play therapist, find ways to encourage play in your space. Bring toys, play music, and welcome little ones to actively participate in the counseling journey. Playing is an innate human need. People at all developmental stages need a space to be in the moment without a set course. Babies and young children need play to survive. Adults are not much different.

Play moves us away from seeking specific goals or meeting certain tasks. It is about the here and now with fun and joy. As we engage caregivers in play, we support them to connect with a different part of themselves. For some of us, letting go and being in the moment might come easily. For others, we may need further reflection in noticing our internal world before we can lean deeper. However, this attunement and collaboration with what we, caregivers, and little ones need is the anti-oppressive stance. They need to be present in everything we do.

SUMMARY

Play and play therapy are facilitators of change. When a caregiver experiences a mental health complication, it impacts their capacity for fun and joy. As we work to implement a reflective and relational model, play serves as the bridge to the child's world and language. It can also be a bridge to the caregiver's internal experiences. Providers must explore experiences, meaning, and level of comfort that caregivers have with play before introducing it into the clinical space. Each person carries their own story. Provider observations must be understood through the client's lens. Ramon and Julian's story provides an example of exploring readiness and seeing the power of play on the caregiver–child relationship and the caregiver's mental health.

REFERENCES

Association for Play Therapy. (n.d.). About APT. https://www.a4pt.org/page/AboutAPT

Courtney, J. A. (Ed.). (2020). *Infant play therapy*. Routledge.

Drewes, A. A., & Schaefer, C. E. (2016). The therapeutic powers of play. In K. J. O'Connor, C. E. Schaefer, & L. D. Braverman (Eds.), *Handbook of play therapy* (2nd edition) (pp. 35–60). Wiley.

Guerney, L. (2001). Child-centered play therapy. *International Journal of Play Therapy*, *10*(2), 13–31. https://doi.org/10.1037/h0089477

Harris, J. [Men to Heal]. (2020, October 20). *Pregnancy and infant loss a father's grief* [Video]. YouTube. https://www.youtube.com/watch?v=C8F4D0fN-xY&t=1s

Harvard Center on the Developing Child. (n.d.). Serve and return. https://developing child.harvard.edu/science/key-concepts/serve-and-return/

Landreth, G. L. (2012). *Play therapy: The art of the relationship* (3rd edition). Routledge.

Lee, G. Y., & Kisilevsky, B. S. (2014). Fetuses respond to father's voice but prefer mother's voice after birth. *Developmental Psychobiology*, *56*(1), 1–11. https://doi.org/10.1002/dev.21084

Luyten, P., Nijssens, L., Fonagy, P., & Mayes, L. C. (2017). Parental reflective functioning: Theory, research, and clinical applications. *The Psychoanalytic Study of the Child*, *70*(1), 174–199. https://dx.doi.org/10.1080/00797308.2016.1277901

Mota, C., Sánchez, C., Carreño, J., & Gómez, M. E. (2023). Paternal experiences of perinatal loss – A scoping review. *International Journal of Environmental Research and Public Health*, *20*(6), 4886. https://doi.org/10.3390/ijerph20064886

Nijssens, L., Bleys, D., Casalin, S., Vliegen, N., & Luyten, P. (2018). Parental attachment dimensions and parenting stress: The mediating role of parental reflective functioning. *Journal of Child and Family Studies*, *27*(6), 2025–2036. https://doi.org/10.1007/s10826-018-1029-0

Rowland-Shea, J., & Doshi, S. (2020, July 21). *The nature gap: Confronting racial and economic disparities in the destruction and protection of nature in America*. American Progress. https://www.americanprogress.org/issues/green/reports/2020/07/21/487787/the-nature-gap/

Scarff, J. R. (2019). Postpartum depression in men. *Innovations in Clinical Neuroscience*, *16*(5–6), 11–14.

Scott, K. (2017, June 19). *For children of Color playing outside is both dangerous and necessary*. HuffPost. https://tinyurl.com/3cy6prsy

Tenets Initiative. (2018). Diversity-informed tenets for work with infants, children & families/Principios informados en la diversidad para trabajar con bebés, niños, niñas y familias. Irving Harris Foundation. https://diversityinformedtenets.org/download-the-tenets/

Yogman, M., Garner, A., Hutchinson, J., Hirsh-Pasek, K., Golinkoff, R. M., Committee on Psychosocial Aspects of Child and Family Health, & Council on Communications and Media. (2018). The power of play: A pediatric role in enhancing development in young children. *Pediatrics*, *142*(3), e20182058. https://doi.org/10.1542/peds.2018-2058

CHAPTER ELEVEN

The Caregiver as a Whole Person

Many BIPOC families hold loyalties of secrecy around pain and suffering. Narratives such as *"This is a family issue," "This stays at home,"* or *"No pasa nada"* (loosely translated as "nothing's wrong") are common parts of survival within our communities. When our strengths and vulnerabilities have been used against us by a system of supremacy, keeping things in the family and avoiding the perception of need is a survival tactic. The world is not safe. It is dangerous and chaotic. Yet, healing entails finding pockets of safety and connection. Finding and leaning into these pockets of protection can be a hard ask for people. We become good at serving and caring for others while leaving our own needs behind. For many of us, it is hard to ask for help. When individuals transition to caregiverhood, the sense of vulnerability is much higher than at any other time in life. Our capacity to support the caregiver as a *whole person* entails reaching those parts of them that may be outside awareness, including intergenerational trauma and transmissions of strength. This chapter explores a holistic approach to supporting perinatal caregivers at the individual and collective levels.

AUTONOMY AND THE TRANSITION TO CAREGIVERHOOD

Recognizing the cyclical nature of time, we can say that caregiving can occur in the present, past, and future. In the present, caregiving might involve pregnancies and raising children. When a pregnancy or infant loss is part of a family's story, caregiving might be experienced as taking place in the past and present. The past holds memories, hopes, and pain. The present entails navigating grief and finding ways to honor the loss. The unimaginable pain of losing their child is present daily in many caregivers' hearts. Every moment, celebration, and milestone holds their child's memory. Caregiving in the future might involve preconception or adoption planning and dreams and hopes for the child. A person becomes a caregiver in the context of caring for someone else. Can a caregiver exist separately from their responsibility to their children?

I think about Winnicott's (1965) famous quote, "There is no such thing as an infant, meaning, of course, that whenever one finds an infant one finds maternal care, and without maternal care there would be no infant" (p. 39). In a society where we highly value individualism, I wonder whether an individual truly exists in the sense of being separate from others. Maybe our goal for individuality, significantly as related to parenthood, exacerbates our suffering. We need others from birth to our time of death. Connection helps us thrive. We read books that others have written, share stories told by those who came before us, and seek love and belonging from those around us. Belonging does not happen without facilitators (i.e., friends, loved ones, and colleagues). The caregiver learns about themselves, their priorities, and desires in each developmental stage of their life journey.

We re-shift our desires for rest, love, connection, laughter, and protection throughout our lives. Autonomy intertwines with the caregiver's identity. A balanced sense of independence recognizes interconnection in that some choices come from our internal desires while others are the outcomes of things outside ourselves (Chirkov, 2008), like the importance of the collective. As humans, we are constantly negotiating between internal and external needs. Balance helps us survive. My training in perinatal mental health allowed me to shift how I saw and held caregivers in counseling. We are holding space for the complex shifts the individual is experiencing. There is the grief in what no longer will be an option. For example, most caregivers of babies and toddlers cannot just get into their car on a whim at midnight to buy a snack from the corner store.

Similarly, getting ready for the morning is no longer rolling out of bed and heading out ten minutes later. These are fundamental, everyday shifts that can chip away at well-being. People can begin feeling helpless when they experience back-to-back changes to their autonomy in a society that does not support these new developments. When we couple those changes with traumatic experiences and systemic barriers, the load is heavier.

A SPACE BETWEEN FANTASY AND REALITY

Our role is to support people in seeing the fantasy and the reality. The illusion can manifest in an utter sense of helplessness and hopelessness for the future. It can be the space where we start to believe that nothing will ever be the same and interpret that as bad or negative. The fantasy is also the story we tell ourselves about what caregiverhood will be. If the perinatal story we believe is *"This will be the happiest time of my life,"* and then we experience a traumatic birth, an infidelity, or a colicky baby, we might start to tell ourselves that we are a failure. As we partner with clients, we support them in validating the sadness for what is not present and building space for reality. The reality entails seeing what is in front of us with all the complex and messy parts. Life changes when we add a child into our home. Freedom to move around the world has a before and an after when people become caregivers. Survival can push us into an all-or-nothing lens, blurring our capacity to maintain some balance in our perspective. In this case, balance can look like recognizing the moment's difficulty and exploring what we need.

Another example of a fantasy is negating our feelings and needs as humans. People react to changes and stressors in life. Sometimes, people can get stuck and fight with themselves over the belief that they *should* not be distressed when painful situations happen. The internal fight to not feel is reinforced when we come from families and communities that push us to be strong and handle things independently. Unspoken messages and expectations do not always make sense and can create chaos in our inner world. The counseling relationship facilitates understanding of internal conflict and patterns outside awareness. Latin American culture tends to be family-oriented, often believing that problems are resolved within the family. At the same time, my culture upholds *marianismo*, a patriarchal social script that sees women and mothers as all-giving, all-sacrificing, and all-understanding (Castillo et al., 2010). Marianismo's message is, *"Do not complain and do not ask for help because motherhood is your duty."* Many communities hold similar versions of this message where the family is essential, but some members are not allowed permission to ask for help. Our familial, social, and internal scripts can create a barrier to accessing care. Another challenge arises when providers are not finding ports of entry to explore these scripts and their discrepancies.

SITTING WITH GRIEF

Societal and familial messages about the meaning of caregiverhood, mothering, birthing, and fathering can affect our capacity to recognize our present pain. The transition to parenthood is neither inherently bad nor entirely good. It is difficult for most people. To sit with the reality of now requires moving through grief. By leaning into reflection, providers can support the client's capacity to mourn those aspects of themselves that are no longer present. Caregivers are making peace with the transition as both rewarding and imperfect. Grief is required to move through acceptance of the present moment and welcome what is to come. Clients mourn what used to be. The aspects that need mourning during the perinatal period can be broad. For instance, people might also mourn their childhood or the relationship with their parents that they did not have. It is about creating mental space to sit with the person's internal experience. Recognizing our inner world is a gateway to building a relationship with what life can look like moving forward. I find that sometimes providers, especially child therapists, can experience concern about the idea of bringing up the sad parts of being a parent. We care deeply about the children we support and might worry that we cannot provide enough support. It can be difficult as a provider to hear things like, *"I hate being a parent," "I should have never had kids,"* or *"I hate my child."* However, a failure to name taboos around the difficulties and maybe ugly parts of caregiverhood can hinder the person's transition to parenthood.

We can support a sense of balanced autonomy among perinatal people by exploring desires that are still present for them.

- What do they like?
- What activities do they enjoy doing?
- What do they want out of life?
- What is important to them?
- What lights up their world?
- How are they making sense of autonomy during this period in their lives?
- How are early experiences showing up in their relationship to being a caregiver?
- What stories are they telling themselves about their life and future?

REFLECTION PAUSE 1

As you think about your clinical training and life experience:

- How do you think about grief during the transition to parenthood? If you notice discomfort, can you sit with it and wonder what it is trying to tell you and how this experience might be for the caregiver?

  _____
  _____
  _____

- How might a person's upbringing and culture impact their capacity to mourn the transition to parenthood?

  _____
  _____
  _____

THE WHOLE PERSON

Applying a holistic approach through an anti-oppressive lens entails looking at Indigenous ways of being. Terry Cross, the founding executive director of the National Indian Child Welfare Association (NICWA), developed the relational worldview model, a framework for understanding the whole person both individually and collectively (Cross, 1997). In his 1997 paper, *"Understanding relational worldview in Indian families,"* Cross discussed the difference between linear and relational worldviews. The linear view holds a cause-and-effect approach. Cross provided the example of how a Western approach to mental healthcare is about figuring out a diagnosis to provide treatment. The diagnosis is the cause of the symptoms, and if we understand it we can effectively treat the concern. This familiar approach to care can relieve people while alienating many. At the same time, it limits the practitioner's understanding of other factors that impact humans.

The relational worldview stems from Indigenous knowledge and awareness of the cyclical nature of life (Cross, 1997, 2007). It acknowledges that multiple factors impact health and well-being: The context in which we live, our mind, body, and spirit. These aspects have an interrelated relationship within us. The context in which we live entails access to privilege and the barriers we face. The body includes our physical health and things like rest and genetics. The mind speaks to the emotional space and our cognitive world. Gestational and non-gestational caregivers experience significant brain and hormonal changes impacting memory, decision-making, sensitivity, mood, and other caregiving behaviors (Abraham et al., 2014; Kim et al., 2014). The spiritual sphere involves how we create meaning, our relationship to what we consider sacred, and the messages we collect throughout life, both positive and negative, regarding spirituality. The transition to parenthood elicits existential changes such as value systems, the meaning of life, and awareness of mortality (Prinds et al., 2021). When one of the four features is not in balance, well-being declines. A lack of harmony in one or more factors can lead to suffering. When a perinatal mental health complication comes into a family, it shifts the balance and changes the social context. People can suffer without support in creating harmony within those factors, often in silence. Many things disrupt the balance. For instance, the hormonal shifts people experience during pregnancy, delivery, and the postnatal period, coupled with disruption from systemic barriers and intergenerational trauma, will trigger imbalance in the four quadrants.

THE HOLISTIC JOURNEY

A holistic approach that is anti-oppressive takes into consideration the different aspects of a person. Holistic frameworks move beyond mind and body to include a connection to spirituality and the collective. As we think about expanding our way of working to truly support diverse populations, we must consider the meaning of healing and liberation for ourselves and the communities we support. Our definitions and ways of understanding others require constant assessment because everyone we encounter is different. Each experience is unique. The unexamined parts of our privilege make the barriers others experience invisible to us. Dominant narratives have and continue to vilify practices that bring healing and strength to many members of the global majority. When our communities were colonized, we were told that our healing, medicine, and connection to Spirit were evil. Many of us lost a link to our cultures of origin and practices. Dominant mental health discourses can disparage those of us who connect or are in the process of reconnecting with our ancestral traditions. Providers and the healthcare system at large can unintentionally minimize the importance of spiritual healing. They can trivialize practices by appropriating and reselling them to us under a whitewashed lens. Take, for example, the importance of nature. Indigenous communities have been caring for the land since time immemorial. Many fields are now coming to terms with the benefits of breathing fresh air and spending time with plants and trees. What do we do as a result? We commodified nature as another way to sell a product (i.e., capitalism), with little respect for honoring Indigenous ways of being that hold this sacred knowledge. This journey is not about purchasing another training. It is about learning how to be with ourselves and with others.

Moving through an anti-oppressive way of being requires constantly analyzing how the past impacts this present moment and our discourses. Those with higher access to privilege hold a different experience and perspective than those placed on the margins by structural racism and colonization. Tenet 1, our self-awareness, remains our compass to partnering with others (Tenets Initiative, 2018). It is how we learn where to move in session with a client, what trainings to engage in, and from whom to seek learning and mentoring. We will not find a perfect training, book, or person, but we can strive to hold a critical lens to everything we learn. We can wonder about the skills we do not have and what that means to our relationship with our implicit biases. A technique here is that when you notice a strong feeling regarding a therapeutic skill or framework, ask yourself what that means and where it is coming from. This practice will come in handy as we discuss ancestral healing, connection to Spirit or Source, dreams, nature, and other soul-based ways of being throughout this chapter (and throughout life because, hopefully, our learning will continue as long as we have breath).

We will not know what each unique need is for everyone we meet. People come to us from all walks of life with immense pain. When they do not hear themselves reflected in our identities and practices, we unintentionally contribute to a barrier to access to care. Taking a full-person approach to counseling perinatal people helps us create an access point to their world. We are not going to be experts in everything. My ask for readers is consistent throughout this text: Can we meet people in a w–ay that is attuned to their needs?

BEYOND THE DOMINANT LENS

The Tenet "Recognize and respect non-dominant bodies of knowledge" steers providers towards knowing that different people have many ways to find strength, heal, and understand the world (Tenets Initiative, 2018, para. 4). Evidenced-based practice is part of an extensive network of resources people have been tapping into since the beginning of time. It is not *one* ultimate answer for all communities. No one way of being can be the answer to wellness for all. Moving beyond colonial-based practices requires constantly acknowledging the wisdom present in each person. Each human is a knowledge holder, bringing gifts into the client–therapist relationship. Providers know human development, evidenced-based practices, and hold skills for strategically partnering with others. We also have our history, ancestral knowledge, and inner wisdom. The individuals we work with are no different. We will not know their gifts until we begin working with them, but we need to recognize that they bring wisdom, knowledge, experience, and strengths that enrich our work, their families, and our world. Critical thinking is one way to maintain a connection with our constant need to balance dominant with nondominant knowledge. Dominant ways of being put us into the role of an expert who guides and empowers the client. Critiquing, shifting, and expanding our clinical knowledge are means to move away from the dominant role in the counseling relationship (St. John et al., 2012). Those strategies help us see the soul of this work and the others in our collaboration. Failure to see our role as a collaborator in care increases the risk of harm to the clients we aim to support.

REFLECTION PAUSE 2

Please take a moment to reflect, write, or draw upon these questions. As you think about supporting the individual perinatal person:

- What are the clinical skills that you bring?

  _____
  _____
  _____

- How does the delivery of those skills align with non-dominant ways of being?

  _____
  _____
  _____

- What non-dominant ways inform your practice?

  _____

  _____

  _____

- What comes up when you consider critiquing, shifting, and expanding interventions?

  _____

  _____

  _____

- What barriers do you face as a provider that may inhibit your capacity to change the way you practice?

  _____

  _____

  _____

- How can you negotiate with those barriers in a way that still recognizes and respects different forms of healing?

  _____

  _____

  _____

HEALING AND THE RELATIONAL WORLDVIEW

Consider how the relational worldview applies to your work. I often move between wanting to throw away all my past training and Westernized ways of being and honoring that everything I learned is a gift that made me into who I am today. All you learned and experienced helped create the responsive, caring, and critically reflective clinician you are today. Our training and skills are vital to supporting communities and, at the same time, have intrinsic limitations. We are holding those truths and the reality that there is always something we can do differently to examine how implicit biases impact our understanding of the human experience, pathology, and treatment. The relational worldview helps us embody Tenet 8, the allocation of resources to systems of change (Tenets Initiative, 2018). We are the most excellent resource we have. Learning, reflecting, and stretching past our comfort zone can be a tool to dismantle oppression in our work and promote belonging to the clients we support and the clinicians we may supervise.

Mind

The mind realm encompasses our intellectual and emotional center. Our intellect helps us learn, grow, and connect (Cross, 2007). The emotional center is a space to understand our values, traditions, identities, emotional states, and perhaps connection with others. Although many individuals do not have traumatic experiences in childhood, all of us have human caregivers. Caregivers who made mistakes, missed cues, and did not meet our every need. As a whole, the perinatal period and caregiverhood stir up the wounds of relationships with our family of origin. Conceptualizing the needs of the perinatal individual entails understanding what they carry from the past and how it makes sense in the present context. If a caregiver is experiencing feelings of inadequacy, we want to know whether these feelings connect to something from an earlier life event/experience or ancestral wound. Inadequacy can come from the direct and subtle messages that others give regarding our capacity.

Immigrants and children of immigrants are often residing in between cultures, confronting, making sense, and navigating the values from their cultures of origin and those from the dominant frame. Growing up in a community where praising children is not the norm might require an examination of our self-view when one becomes a caregiver. Isabelle Allende, one of my favorite novelists, wrote in her book *The soul of a woman* (2021) that she grew up and raised children in a community where getting good grades and winning were just the expectations. There was no praise for good behavior. Allende explained that her children pushed back on her parenting value system as they became parents, considering it rigid and disconnected. All humans must navigate the space between *how things used to be done* and *how it is now*. Many examples come to mind as I think about the shifting of worldview. I will share some perinatal family stories below with examples of reflective questions I ask myself. Please consider these questions and others that may come up as you go through each description.

- **The immigrant perinatal caregiver who believed that parenthood would fulfill their sense of womanhood, who then experiences perineal trauma leading to incontinence**. Amara is a 26-year-old Guatemalan woman who recently delivered her first baby, 3-month-old Karla. Amara grew up in a close and religious family she described as supportive. She married her partner, Allen, two years ago. Amara reported dreaming of motherhood since she was a young child. She planned for a home delivery with a midwife. However, Amara was rushed to hospital after several hours due to no progress to cervical dilation and the risks for the baby. The physician performed a midline episiotomy at the hospital without sharing possible risks or asking for the client's consent. Amara remains in significant pain, experiences incontinence, and has trouble controlling bowel movements.

  How can I partner with this individual to understand the impact of the trauma on their life now and how they view themselves? How does this impact relationships? Sex? Career? Finances? And everything else? As we formulate treatment, how am I considering the implications of the perineal trauma on barriers and privilege? What assumptions am I making about the individual's life and views?

- **The parent who was hit as a child and is now navigating what corporal punishment meant to them as they were growing up and what it means now**. Maria, 33 years old, is raising her 13-month-old nephew, Miguel. Last week Maria kissed Miguel, and he bit her on the lip. Her initial reaction was to hit him in the mouth. Luisa, Miguel's grandmother, observed the interaction and stated, *"See, that's what you get for biting."* Maria reported feeling guilty about hitting him but confused about her mother's reaction. Maria tearfully shared seeing the sadness in Miguel's face and remembering how scared she was of her parents when growing up.

  I want to know how Maria views her relationship with her mother. How close are they? Have they talked about corporal punishment before? What was the intensity and the frequency of the hits Maria received when growing up? Did they leave marks and bruises, both physically and emotionally? Was this the first time she hit Miguel? Does Maria have access to other ways of redirecting toddler behavior? How does Maria cope with stress? How does she understand the guilt she is feeling? For instance, is the guilt's intensity reasonable to this incident or all-consuming? She saw her fear and maybe sadness reflected in Miguel's face after she hit him. Can she hold on to that awareness? How can her engagement guide the journey of being a loving caregiver to herself?

- **The caregiver who was taught that children should cry it out to not get spoiled and is navigating knowing what is best for their baby while getting pressure from others to go against their gut**. Pierre, 24 years old, lives with his mother, aunt, and 5-month-old daughter, Darline. Pierre enjoys carrying and body feeling his baby. His mother and aunt laugh at him as they see him falling asleep while pumping on the couch. His mother says, *"That baby is going to run all over you. You're creating a monster."* Pierre reported needing a full-time job but is concerned that if his mother takes care of Darline, she will let the baby cry until she falls asleep. He is unable to afford a different childcare arrangement. Pierre feels like he is losing a part of himself and failing at life. He has to choose between leaving Darline at home with his family or not making money.

  Pierre is in a tough spot, having limited choices available. Some caregivers can feel like nothing they do is good enough. I wonder how his mother and aunt's criticism impacted his self-view. What about the trust in his capacity to be an effective caregiver to his child? Considering the possibility of a generational and cultural divide, is there a way for Pierre to partner with his mother and aunt?

- **The child who was told nothing they did was ever good enough and is now an adult responsible for the physical and emotional well-being**

of another life. Tamika is five months postpartum, living at home with her baby and partner, Ranya. Tamika reported a history of emotional and physical abuse by her mother. She participated in counseling in the past to address the trauma but notices herself having nightmares about her mother. Tamika has been crying herself to sleep every night for the past three weeks. She has been ruminating about not being good enough and questions whether she can care for her daughter. For the past day, Tamika has been thinking about running away, as she feels the baby will be better off with anyone but her.

I worry about Tamika's well-being. Early childhood trauma leaves a hole inside of us. One that never gets fully filled. It needs attention and care. When significant changes happen in our lives, the pit of childhood trauma can open up, swallowing everything around it. Joy and celebration can turn into sadness and despair. The pain of the past multiplies the challenges people face in early caregiving. I wonder what Tamika's relationship with the pain of childhood trauma has been throughout her life. How aware had she been of the ripples of that pain before her baby joined the family? How was her mental world before pregnancy and delivery? Can she still tap into her capacity to survive?

Physical

The physical quadrant goes beyond our connection to our bodies to how connected one is to a sense of safety. With this lens, we explore how systemic barriers impact access to affordable housing, transportation, healthcare, childcare, and all the other items families need to survive. Our current social context affects well-being in this quadrant. Colonization and systemic racism are present in every aspect of safety. Housing offers more than protection from the elements. It might be the place to build memories and connect with ourselves and our families. When families are supportive, they can be like an oasis in the desert, helping to quench our thirst for connection and our wounds from exposure to the elements. Connection to a supportive family is a privilege that many of us do not have. When this is the case, how are we partnering with clients to find support that makes sense for them? Coming to terms with reality is a painful path to healing. An issue often appearing in counseling is people's fantasy-based expectations of others. Most of the time, the hope fueling the fantasy arises from the desire to be treated with basic human decency. We want family members to respect our decisions, to listen to us, to want to spend time with our children, and maybe even to love us. However, this can be an unrealistic expectation of people who consistently give us the opposite. The healing of the perinatal person includes accepting the reality of what is present in our lives to create space for something else. We get to decide and make what "the something else" will look like.

When a person can accept that their family of origin will/may never be what they need, they can better see when they recreate situations in hopes that their families can love, accept, or see them as worthy. When the re-enactment of dysfunctional patterns comes into awareness, we can protect ourselves from disappointment and all the complex feelings that come with that. Then, we can build on our capacity to find what we need from places that meet that desire. Inequity will continue to impact access to meeting needs, even when we are not re-enacting. What changes is that we are no longer knocking on a door that will not open. For example, suppose I can accept that my family member always says they will give me a ride and typically cancels last minute. In that case, I can bypass asking them and arrange another form of transportation. This seemingly simple change on the outside is about the inner shift in learning to care for ourselves. The therapist guides the client to see what is already within them. Therapists can help clients recognize their capacity to be loving caregivers to themselves and to obtain internal safety in a way that makes sense for them. Complete security is never possible, as the world is dangerous. For instance, in this example, I might still need to figure out public transportation while fearing being sexually harassed (a reality for many survivors), living in a city with a poor transportation system, and enduring terrible weather conditions. However, our capacity to make protective decisions for ourselves increases with awareness, support, and action.

How are we exploring physical safety with clients throughout treatment? Caregiving requires protection. What resources does the individual have to bring security into their lives? Building an internal and family refuge entails connecting with what is available. If others have yet to be reliable, how do we partner with the client to support them in becoming loyal to themselves? A conversation I bring into counseling is the idea of avoiding self-betrayal. This type of betrayal happens when we go against what we want or need to do to please others. Families with babies and young children receive constant opinions about what they should be doing. If a perinatal caregiver is having trouble resting and wants to co-sleep to avoid getting out of bed, I need to put my training on safe sleep aside to be of support. Co-sleeping is a way for the caregiver to establish physical safety in this example.

Spirituality

Our final stop in this exploration is Spirit and the sacred. Most people who access mental health services value spirituality and benefit from having it integrated into their care (Yamada et al., 2020). Spirituality was the most ignored quadrant in my mental health training. I often equated spirituality with organized religion, which became a wall to expanding my thinking. I had to engage in a lot of reflection, supervision, and training (dominant and non-dominant) to dig deep into my understanding of this part of human experience. Understanding our inner world helps create space within us to hold the internal stories of another. Let us engage in some reflection before continuing.

REFLECTION PAUSE 3

- What does spirituality mean to you?

  _____

  _____

  _____

- What do you need to support someone whose definition of spirituality differs from yours?

  _____

  _____

  _____

- How does spirituality show up in how you live?

  _____

  _____

  _____

- How does it show up in your work with clients and communities?

  _____

  _____

  _____

Spirituality will look different for each person. It might mean a connection with the purpose of our lives, Spirit, Source, God, Goddess, higher self, nature, peace, self-love, community, or anything else that the person brings. We must follow the client's lead in exploring what spirituality means to them, their source of strength or hope, or what brings calm to their lives. We want to explore the deeper meaning of rituals and practices that the client may have. Rituals and practices can include prayer, meditation, time in nature, singing, smoke cleansing, working with a spiritual guide, exploring dreams, setting up a shrine, making offerings, and lighting candles. We must intentionally ask specific questions and give examples to establish that all spirituality is welcome in the clinical space. Colonized communities had their traditional practices stolen from them and replaced with Westernized belief systems. Many grew up believing that anything outside the dominant lens was evil. Even if we did not receive that exact message at home, evidenced-based interventions abound in the mental health field.

The intersection of mental health and spirituality carries a unique perspective on stigma. The stigma surrounding mental health issues has long hindered open discussions and acceptance. Take a client who communicates with spirits and hears and sees things others do not: Does our mind jump to the possibility of a psychotic disorder? Or are we open to exploring the strengths of their practices to their well-being? Spirituality often gives individuals a sense of meaning, purpose, and connection. A strong sense of purpose can contribute to better mental health by providing a framework for understanding one's place in the world, the challenges we face, and the strengths available.

Many messages impacting how we see ourselves have been with us and our loved ones throughout the generations. Black and Brown communities survived unimaginable traumas. The scars of those experiences can remain present in how we navigate the world. Another truth about this life is that none of us come out unscathed. We hold stories of survival and pain from our lineages. Healing the collective is about the connections we make with others in our lifetime and the internal world we carry. We stand on the love of our ancestors, those who came before us. They are present in how we experience and navigate the world. We might develop internal relationships with different parts of our ancestors. These relationships might be based on memories, stories we hear, or our imagination (Dennison & Powell-Watts, 2021). We may carry deep ancestral wounds when deep intergenerational trauma is part of our story. It can be hard to connect to ancestral strength.

Ancestral healing is an approach that recognizes the interconnectedness between our past, present, and future generations. It involves acknowledging and addressing the emotional, psychological, and spiritual wounds passed down through family lines. We can integrate this work in counseling in different ways, such as asking directly about ancestors, exploring internal object relations, doing shadow work, and practicing visualization and guided imagery. We will never be fully competent in everything; the key here is practicing from a place of humility where we lean with the client into their unknown. We want enough flexibility to expand and hold what shows up for the person. Additional training, reflective supervision, community discussion, and critical self-reflection support breaking from rigid practice patterns.

Context

The context quadrant reminds us that everything is connected. One thing impacts the other. Understanding the perinatal experience requires an individual and a collective lens. This quadrant refers to how systems of oppression affect the individual, social, political, and ecological environments we may navigate at three levels (Cross, 1997):

- Micro: The individual caregiver's values, beliefs, experiences, and close relationships.

- Mezzo: Familial relationships, neighborhood, work, school, providers, and environment.
- Macro: This level includes systems like financial, housing, transportation, medical, political, and legal.

Collaborating with clients entails examining how access to resources, safety, and opportunities impact overall well-being for them and their families (Cross, 2007). We can also examine how connection to culture and intergenerational strengths impacts wellness.

How do we consider context as we conceptualize treatment strategies? Let us take the example of support groups, as they are a helpful source of connection for the perinatal period. Their accessibility entails access to some forms of privilege, such as the capacity to attend, whether in person or telehealth. Transportation, time, protection from the elements, and a sense of safety can impact a person's ability to participate in in-person meetings. Meanwhile, access to reliable technology and privacy are added concerns for attending a telehealth group. Additionally, as providers, are we examining the goodness of fit for the person and the group? Am I unintentionally sending an individual to a group where no one looks and thinks like them? How did I partner with the client to examine whether a support group would be a good fit? For instance, did we discuss other resources within their communities that the client might be interested in?

SUMMARY

Life, values, needs, and desires constantly shift during pregnancy and postpartum. Perinatal people are in a constant state of transition. A balanced sense of autonomy entails grieving the changes to independence when a baby joins a family. An anti-oppressive way of supporting perinatal people involves a holistic care approach. Providers lean on the relational worldview model and take a whole-person approach to working with perinatal people (Cross, 2007). This model examines the interrelation between well-being and the four quadrants: context, mind, physical, and spiritual.

REFERENCES

Abraham, E., Hendler, T. Shapira-Lichter, I., Kanat-Maymon, Y., Zagoory-Sharon, O., & Feldman, R. (2014). Father's brain is sensitive to childcare experiences. *Proceeding from the National Academy of Sciences*, *111*(27), 9792–9797. https://doi.org/10.1073/pnas.1402569111

Allende, I. (2021). *The soul of a woman*. Random House.

Castillo, L. G., Perez, F. V., Castillo, R., & Ghosheh, M. R. (2010). Construction and initial validation of the Marianismo Beliefs Scale. *Counselling Psychology Quarterly*, *23*(2), 163–175. https://doi.org/10.1080/09515071003776036

Chirkov, V. I. (2008). Culture, personal autonomy and individualism: Their relationships and implications for personal growth and well-being. In G. Zheng, K. Leung, & J. G. Adair (Eds.), *Perspectives and progress in contemporary cross-cultural psychology: Proceedings from the 17th International Congress of the International Association for Cross-Cultural Psychology*. https://scholarworks.gvsu.edu/cgi/viewcontent.cgi?article=1127&context=iaccp_papers

Cross, T. L. (1997). Understanding relational worldview in Indian families. *Pathways Practice Digest*, *12*(4).

Cross, T. L. (2007, September 20). Through Indigenous eyes: Rethinking theory and practice. Paper presented at the 2007 *Conference of the Secretariat of Aboriginal and Islander Child Care in Adelaide*, Australia.

Dennison, A., & Powell-Watts, L. (2021). Ancestral healing in psychotherapy. *Spirituality in Clinical Practice*, *8*(3), 188–194. https://doi.org/10.1037/scp0000254

Kim, P., Rigo, P., Mayes, L. C., Feldman, R., Leckman, J. F., & Swain, J. E. (2014). Neural plasticity in fathers of human infants. *Social Neuroscience*, *9*(5), 522–535. https://doi.org/10.1080/17470919.2014.933713

Prinds, C., Timmerman, C., Hvidtjørn, D., Ammentorp, J., Christian Hvidt, N., Larsen, H., & Toudal Viftrup, D. (2021). Existential aspects in the transition to parenthood based on interviews and a theatre workshop. *Sexual & Reproductive Healthcare*, *28*, 100612. https://doi.org/10.1016/j.srhc.2021.100612

St. John, S. M., Thomas, C., & Noroña, C. R. (2012). Infant mental health professional development: Together in the struggle for social justice. *Zero to Three Journal*, *33*(2), 13–22.

Tenets Initiative. (2018). Diversity-informed tenets for work with infants, children & families/Principios informados en la diversidad para trabajar con bebés, niños, niñas y familias. Irving Harris Foundation. https://diversityinformedtenets.org/download-the-tenets/

Winnicott, D. W. (1965). *The maturational processes and the facilitating environment: Studies in the theory of emotional development*. Karnac.

Yamada, A.-M., Lukoff, D., Lim, C. S. F., & Mancuso, L. L. (2020). Integrating spirituality and mental health: Perspectives of adults receiving public mental health services in California. *Psychology of Religion and Spirituality*, *12*(3), 276–287. https://doi.org/10.1037/rel0000260

Transitioning Out of Counseling

CHAPTER TWELVE

The Therapeutic Pause

Healing is a lifelong journey. The path has twists, turns, and some roadblocks along the way. We can overcome some barriers alone but require relationships to survive or push through others. With the proper support, each step we take brings us closer to a connection with ourselves and our loved ones. The perinatal period is unique. Caregivers and their children face significant vulnerability. Babies depend solely on those around them to care for them, while caregivers also need others' holding and support. We live in a society with policies and ideals that do not support the well-being of families. Although we define the perinatal period as the time between pregnancy and the first two years postpartum, the need for relational healing does not stop throughout life. We need each other for survival. We think of the therapeutic relationship as having a beginning, middle, and end. In my experience, the demands of pregnancy, postpartum, and babyhood make perinatal treatment shorter term than most other forms of care. However, because life is complex and relationships heal, I like to think about concluding treatment as a pause rather than as a final endpoint. A counseling break leaves the door open for returning if and when it is needed. This chapter explores the therapeutic pause and strategies for the end stage of care.

A STORY ABOUT ENDS

Working in the mental health system is tough, for many different reasons. Providers face the challenge of navigating problematic systems and complex relationships with colleagues and supervisors. In my journey, the clinical work of psychotherapy and supervision has consistently been rewarding more times than not. Relationships with clients teach and change us when we are willing to listen. Terminating counseling services with clients was one of the most complex parts of working in community mental health. The first time I closed with a client hit me so hard that I cried all the way home after the visit. I imagined it would be difficult, but I was not ready for the flood of emotions that washed over me like a tsunami. I felt ashamed and did not want to confide in my supervisor. I was concerned about being unprofessional by being too sensitive and over-connected with clients. Fear of how our colleagues and supervisors view us is one of the reasons why we may not seek help when needed. At least, it was for me. I hid my vulnerable parts until I felt safe enough to lean into my insecurities with a supervisor (and a therapist) I trusted. Part of the intensity of my emotions at that first termination was due to my healing journey, while the other related to the closeness of the clinical relationship. We care deeply about the people we support. This work is heart-and-soul work. We carry clients' stories and feelings within us. We cheer, worry, laugh, and stress for and with them. The end of the therapeutic relationship can feel like a psychic death. The person is still alive, but you can no longer reach them. I wish this idea was enough justification for the systems that decide a client no longer meets the criteria for care without thoroughly assessing their needs. Those of us who might have been in situations where we suddenly lost connection with clients know the pain and uncertainty of that moment.

Over the past 14 years, I have transitioned from many clinical jobs. Each subsequent termination with clients has been challenging for me, even when prepared and supported. One system I try to implement is the idea that the therapeutic relationship can terminate or pause and continue later. We can break care as needed and desired by the client. For instance, most perinatal clients work with me for six months to a year. People sometimes rush recovery due to the demands of caregiverhood and the barriers an oppressive system imposes on them. Even when meeting via telehealth, coming to therapy requires a certain amount of financial and emotional bandwidth. When symptoms decrease, people often find they are busy and must step away. Paying for counseling or making time for it can be emotionally taxing. I think of mental health services as a regular part of healthcare. Yet, I know that we need different things depending on our experiences and capacity at each moment. A client might have enough time for *good enough* care until panic attacks decrease during the first pregnancy and be ready for longer term depth counseling on their second pregnancy or at another time. I support this flexibility for them and for me. I leave the door open to continually return to work together or with another provider when needed. People know that I may not have the same time or immediate availability, but it works for us for the most part.

I practice this way because it is hard to retell our stories repeatedly to different providers. It is a way to honor the relationship and the highs and lows of life. I am free to work this way, as I am in private practice. This flexibility is unavailable for many in community mental health or other clinical settings. I partner with organizations with a similar frame where clinicians are welcome to continue therapeutic relationships after exiting our program. This frame is one of the ways we train student interns and clinicians in our clinical program at Perinatal Support Washington. Sometimes, providers and organizations can unintentionally (and intentionally) get stuck in a cycle of scarcity mindset and competitiveness. This competitiveness can cloud how we think and do our work. We might end up creating arbitrary policies within organizations that can serve to uphold white supremacy. An example that comes to mind is non-compete contracts for providers. It reminds me of the white supremacy characteristics of individualism and power hoarding (see Chapter 5). There are enough potential therapy clients worldwide, and people are not properties. The more we support each other, the better for our communities. I invite you to think about the Tenet, "Advance Policy That Supports All Families," as you consider policies in your organization as related to clinicians and overall client care (Tenets Initiative, 2018, para. 10). Here is a question to reflect on as you write, review, amend, or vote on policy: How does this advance justice, equity, and liberation for families?

If your clinical relationship is coming to the end of its chapter, reflective supervision/consultation can offer providers support as they hold clients. If you are an organization leader, consider this type of supervision or consultation for your team (See Chapter 5). The best way to support clients is to nurture providers. Can we move towards a systemic shift where we support clinicians to give from overflow instead of reserves? Overwhelm, burnout, and compassion fatigue are common in our work. Colonization and structural racism create barriers for providers and for those we want to support. Clinicians newest to the field often support individuals with the most risk and need. While this is a reality that we will not change in one day, there is still work that we can do today, tomorrow, and the days after to create positive and impactful changes.

SUPPORTING THE TRANSITION

Many do not get the space and support to compassionately transition clients out of therapy. Whether you implement a termination model or a treatment pause as a frame (something I recognize is not realistic for many of us), preparation between the therapist and the client is essential. A past professor used to say to the class in our MSW program, *"Termination begins in the first session."* Many of us have heard versions of this message throughout our training. I wish I remembered the professor's name or which class it was, because the words have stayed with me throughout my career. Clients must be provided with enough information to know that ending or pausing is part of the therapy (Vasquez et al., 2008). When treatment is time-limited, the first step is to let the client know that an ending will happen. This conversation must go beyond a brief mention at intake or a sentence in the consent documentation. Providers can dedicate time to this conversation at the beginning of care so that the client can truly give informed consent before deciding to share their story and build a relationship with us.

Time-Limited Care

If you, the organization you work with, or the entity paying for the client's services (insurer/grantor) has time-limited care, think about how you create space for informed consent related to the length of treatment. How are you holding those conversations with clients during the beginning, middle, and end of care?

At the beginning of care, we can explore the client's needs and ensure they are appropriate for what we can offer during our time together. Let us look at an example. Manuel, a client seeking support for perinatal obsessive-compulsive disorder (OCD), trouble bonding with their child, and a history of significant developmental trauma, seeks counseling from a program that provides nine months of care. Given the limited timeframe, we will likely not have the time to work on all concerns. Setting realistic expectations around treatment goals can be a way to remember how much time we have together. During the beginning stages, the therapists let Manuel know the program's timeframe and explore goals the client wants to prioritize. Once they reach the middle of their time together, the provider can review progress and explore what they will focus on for the remainder of the time. The therapist can invite the client to examine progress and discuss the next steps. At four months into care, Manuel reported experiencing relief in OCD symptoms. During the progress review conversation, Manuel shared that he wanted to work on his relationship with his child. He reported understanding that we might not have time to focus on some of the trauma he experienced in childhood. In the seventh month, the therapist began exploring the possibility of referrals and more frequently discussing their time left in counseling.

One of the challenges in time-limited care is that time passes quickly, and we can forget that the client will need a reminder that sessions will end soon. If the conversations are not happening throughout treatment, termination might be trickier. Let us return to the ending care as being a psychic death. Discussing the termination close to the end with minimal mentions of it before can leave the client in shock. It does not allow time for preparation. It tends to stir up old feelings, fears, and memories of abandonment. Keeping the end in mind maintains a collaborative relationship. Many situations can impact the capacity to continue sessions: The client's insurance provider might change, they might move out of state, or begin a job with a schedule that does not work with the therapist's availability. The therapeutic relationship might then become time-limited or shorter than previously discussed.

A scenario that is likely common for many providers is switching jobs or transitioning to a different role within the same organization. When we exit an organization or position, we may not have the time to extend termination over several sessions. The reality of a two-week or even a month's notice is that it moves fast. In the time left, we are typically wrapping up documentation, coordinating possible referrals, and trying to schedule sessions before we leave. Self-reflection and consultation usually take a back seat as we complete everything else. The shock of knowing that your therapist is going away and the stirring of attachment wounds that can happen may lead clients to miss or avoid those ending sessions. Endings are complicated, and the likelihood of missing termination sessions is self-protective. Perhaps bringing this idea into session is a way to recognize the closeness of the clinical relationship and the feelings surrounding its end. We might fear that naming the ambivalence that rises towards the end may make the person not come to the ending sessions. I see it as validating the difficulty of the moment and collaborating. It can offer a way for the person to make sense of their feelings. It also communicates that we get it. This moment might hurt. Naming it can also help the provider hold the client with gentleness when they cancel those termination sessions. Here is an example of something we can say to support the transition: *"I know this is coming fast. We will have a chance to talk more during the next two weeks as we wrap up our time. Because endings are tough, you might find yourself not wanting or being unable to make it to our meetings. I hope you come, and I understand if you decide otherwise."*

Taking a Pause

I am a fan of psychodynamic treatment. However, pausing treatment is another divergence from traditional depth psychology frameworks. Clients and I will explore lowering the frequency of our meetings as we move towards a pause. This idea looks like meeting weekly, bi-weekly, monthly, and then pausing until needed. The pause model entails access to making choices for the therapist and client. You can lean on the client, the therapeutic relationship, and your clinical judgment to explore when to change frequency. If a client contacts me two years post-pause to schedule a session and request monthly meetings, I recommend having an appointment before discussing frequency. I might have concerns if a client experiencing high distress requests to meet every other week. I will likely share my hesitation and listen to their feedback. Sometimes, a person may benefit from weekly sessions but can only attend bi-weekly. I need to balance the client's autonomy and my role to provide appropriate care in all instances. It is complex, as an anti-oppressive lens means working to stabilize power hierarchies. I often wonder about the clinical definition of proper care. How does it align with the client's right to self-determination? When I notice parts that do not align with their right to choose, what can I shift to build collaboration in a way that still meets my legal and ethical mandates as a licensed provider? Consultation with other anti-oppressive and reflective practitioners helps me navigate these difficult questions.

Transitioning out of the counseling relationship requires support for the client and the therapist. The termination or treatment pause conversations can extend over several sessions to allow space for reflection and co-creating meaning.

MEANINGFUL ENDS

Conversations, activities, and rituals can serve as ways to honor the therapeutic relationship. Let us pause here to engage in some reflection.

- How do you think about termination?

  _____

  _____

  _____

- What do you notice in your body as you think about it?

  _____

  _____

  _____

- How do you partner with clients during the end of treatment?

  _____

  _____

  _____

- What are your sources of support when endings are difficult?

  _____

  _____

  _____

- What might make a termination challenging regarding cultural differences between the provider and the client?

  _____

  _____

  _____

- How do you create meaning during the last sessions?

_____

_____

_____

The client, the provider, and the relationship will dictate the direction of the ending sessions. Termination is a process, ideally not left to one session. In many cases, conversations about progress, strengths, and any needs that require referrals are enough to support the end stage. If you are seeking more, a helpful strategy for all our work is to ask the client how they would like to create meaning in your last sessions.

The client might have their own sense of what feels like an appropriate ending. Attuning to what they need can help therapists determine if our desire for a ritual or meaning comes from the client's needs or our worry, sadness, or other feelings about ending care. It is about figuring out whether what I am noticing belongs to me, the client, or is something we are co-creating. Is it my worry that I am abandoning the client? Am I re-enacting my fear of abandonment or other similar trauma with the client? Is it the client asking for something more? Or are there patterns we are creating based on the relationship/re-enactment of unconscious material?

I want to understand the client's meaning of our work together for their life and caregiving. A reflective stance to counseling entails exploring this meaning throughout our work together. It is not solely left for the ending stage of treatment. Instead, partnering and collaboration make the work relational. Attention to the relationship and the therapist's constant exploration of the feelings and beliefs that impact care is the secret sauce that deepens the relationship. Our anti-oppressive stance helps guide everything we do. This lens allows us to decipher how our biases might impact conceptualizations. It is the filter for our work and a reminder that biases, instinct, and automatic thoughts are interrelated. The essence of humility is knowing that we will not know everything. Competence is an illusion. We determine the next step by partnering, collaborating, and checking hypotheses with clients.

Here are some ideas you can explore with clients as a starting point for termination activities:

- Sharing a poem in session. You can give the client a copy at the end of your time.
- Sharing a song. It could be a song that you and the client heard together in session or one that speaks to the client's strengths.
- Taking a photo together. A picture with the family can serve as a reminder of the relationship.

- Write a story for the perinatal caregiver and their child. It can be a story about their journey, one with symbolic meaning, or with some loving and respectful touches between the caregiver and their child (hugs, kisses, high-fives).
- Share food. One of my most fun ending sessions involved cake. I do not have a sweet tooth, but there was something special about the caregiver asking their little one how they wanted to say bye. Their child chose a cake party. Food brings communities together. Sharing a meal or treat with others can be nurturing.
- Grow something together. I ran a perinatal group where the ending token was a small culinary herb kit for the families. In session, you can plant something together or share cuttings of plants for propagation for those who enjoy gardening and caring for the earth.
- Share a meditation. The meditation can be a video you found online, a recording you made for the client, or one you wrote up for them.
- Create an art piece. If you integrate expressive strategies into your work, consider painting or creating something with clay. For example, you and the client can create a figure with clay. You can share the process with each other in two ways: (1) You can keep the client's creation, and the client takes yours, or (2) you each keep the one you created as a reminder of your time together.
- Meaningful tokens. I picked up the habit of collecting heart stones from one of my mentors. I like to use them throughout sessions for play or work in the sand tray. They also make tokens to share with clients (and trainees) at the end of our time together. Think about what is meaningful to you and the client. Tokens include small toys (fidgets for the grown-ups and soft ones for the babies), a journal, a small book, affirmation cards, and anything else that makes sense.

Again, the most essential resource we have as providers is ourselves. As long we are critically reflective and collaborative, the end sessions can be meaningful in themselves. We do not need much more than authenticity and presence to create meaning. We can get lost in our thoughts when overplanning. If I hand the client a heart stone at our last meeting and we had never discussed or used stones in counseling, the client might be confused. It does not matter how meaningful heart stones are to me. The token only makes sense with the relational connection. The same goes for all the suggestions above. Many years ago, I went to a training on mindfulness, and the speaker reminded us that we do not need props like scripts, music, or special lighting to be effective. Even as a play therapist who loves a good prop, the trainer's message spoke to the more significant meaning of presence. Our capacity to be in the moment is the agent of change. When in doubt, attune. It has no substitute.

CONSIDERATIONS

Throughout the life of treatment, we will explore concerns, triggers, patterns, and the client's strengths. Sometimes, I notice that as we approach the end, clients may report increased distress or a fear that symptoms have returned. When this happens, it is an opportunity to explore what the client's experience might mean. The thought of an end can stir up feelings of distress and a fear of being alone. One possibility for the distress is that the client might not be ready to end the relationship or lower the frequency of meetings. If we have a choice over this, a remedy is to discuss the client's feelings and explore what they need. When we do not have a choice over extending sessions, having support in place can be helpful.

THE WELLNESS PLAN

The wellness plan (WP) is a tool developed by Perinatal Support Washington (n.d.) for organizing protective factors in a person's life. Clients and providers use the WP as a starting point for guiding care. The WP outlines supportive persons, activities, and ways of thinking that help in times of stress (See Figure 12.1). I want to present the tool in this section as a resource for developing a support plan during treatment pause or termination. As you review the WP, you might find that other areas critical to the client must be included (See an example below). The beauty of anti-oppressive care is that it is individualized. There is not one path nor one set of items that supports all. Ideally, by the time termination happens, we have discussed all the areas of the WP with the client during the life of treatment. Using the WP as a tool for transitioning the client out of care makes termination discussions a review of our work together. Through a relational frame, any post-treatment plan takes a whole-person approach and considers the needs of the caregiver, the child(ren), and any other loved ones who participated in counseling. Focusing on individual needs and relationships helps us move away from a caregiver or child-only approach to therapy.

WP has ideas for each section and explains how to use the form as a tool for wellness (Perinatal Support Washington, n.d.). The following are additional reflective questions to help the client consider the end transition and the relational approach.

Creating a Wellness Plan

Need help completing this plan or finding referrals?
Call Perinatal Support Washington's Warm Line to complete a wellness plan: 1-888-404-7763.

Therapy:
Therapy with a professional experienced in PMADs is crucial to getting better. Detail names, phone numbers, addresses, and next appointments.

Sleep Plan:
Aim for chunks of 4–5 hours of uninterrupted sleep. Detail how to schedule sleep.

Medical Management/Medications:
Medication might be the right decision for you. Detail names of health care providers; appointment details, medication names and dosages.

Other Support Team Members:
Grandparents, sisters, friends, church members, postpartum doula....

Nutrition Plan:
Emphasize protein to improve mood. Detail shopping, meal prep, and food ideas.

Support Group:
Social support is critical to reducing stress and to feel valued and cared for. Detail names, locations and meeting info for local groups.

Me Time/Couple Time:
What things rejuvenate you? Detail when you will have time by yourself and time with just your partner.

Household Help:
What can you delegate? What can you give up for now? List ideas and who will do what.

FIGURE 12.1 Perinatal Support Washington's Wellness Plan

Common Questions About Creating a Wellness Plan

Do I need therapy? How could a therapist or counselor help?
This might be exactly the question that a therapist could answer with you. There are so many things happening to you right now--talking through them would be helpful. A therapist can also offer perspective on whether what you are experiencing is postpartum depression/anxiety/traumatic response, etc. For parents experiencing these issues, a specialist with training and experience is important. Find a therapist near you on our providers list: www.perinatalsupport.org/providers.

What about medications? I've never used them. Will I have to be on them forever? What if I am breastfeeding?
First off, needing/wanting medication is not a weakness, and it may not be the right choice for everyone. Medication is a tool that can be helpful for some and may be needed for others. We highly encourage you to meet with a well-trained provider on this issue, and to use the following sites to learn more: infantrisk.com or womensmentalhealth.org. You can find more resources for medication management on our website, perinatalsupport.org.

I obviously want more sleep, but how? Can sleep deprivation really cause the feelings I am having?
Sleep dramatically impacts our mood, and can be the biggest risk factor for mental health symptoms. Sometimes the very first treatment intervention for depression or anxiety symptoms will be sleep--that's how important it is. A sleep plan is way more than "sleep when the baby sleeps." It entails scheduling shifts with your partner so that you both get good sleep and asking for help to ensure that you are getting a minimum of 4-5 hours of sleep plus shorter stretches throughout the night and day.

A support group--really?
Support groups get a bad rap--maybe we should call them something else. The bottom line is that you will likely be surprised by our groups. They are down-to-earth, refreshingly honest, and often bring some humor to an otherwise difficult time. Also, they are a great way to meet other parents, and they are a great baby/parent-friendly place to go in the first weeks when you just want to get out of the house but haven't mastered breastfeeding in public, are not sure what to bring, etc. We have groups all around the state with times throughout the day and week. Social support is crucial to reducing stress; meeting other parents going through the same life struggles can be the best medicine.

How am I supposed to eat healthy when I can't even find time to eat, let alone cook?
Have you found yourself stuck holding a sleeping baby, without food or water for hours on end? Stash water bottles and healthy snacks on the coffee table. Prepare hardboiled eggs, 12 at a time. Focus on eating high-protein and highly nutrient-rich foods often. These will help balance your blood sugar. Have foods available that you can eat one-handed, such as yogurt, meat, cheese, pre-cut veggies and fruit, or pre-made smoothies from the store. Aim for no cooking, no plates, no utensils (well sometimes)--just open the fridge, grab, and put in your mouth. This phase won't last forever and usually when you're not taking good care of yourself, you feel worse and vice versa. It seems small, but eating well matters.

How can I possibly fit in me time? I'm feeding or attending to my baby all the time.
Taking care of yourself in the first weeks and months can seem like an impossible task, and taking care of your relationship might seem even harder. We strongly encourage you (and your partner) to take time every few days to yourself. This will look very different for each of us. And for many of us, the things we used to do to take care of ourselves are not possible. It's important to think small and schedule time regularly. What brought you joy pre-baby? Here are some ideas: hot shower by yourself, phone a friend, play music that makes you feel good, journal/jot down your thoughts and feelings (sticky notes ok!), or listen to a mindfulness meditation or a podcast.

I'm overwhelmed by the state of my home, and it's stressing me out. How can I get on top of things?
For household help, think of what you can delegate and what you can give up for now. Enlist everyone to do everything you don't want to do. Your job is to rest, heal, and take care of the baby. We mean it! If you don't have someone to ask, let things stay undone. You will get to it--at some point you will need clean dishes and you will do them.

What do you mean by a support team?
Is there someone in your life that you feel comfortable telling it like it is? A friend, a sibling, a parent, a partner? It's important to share how you are really feeling and process this intense experience you have been through. These are the people who you can ask for help, you can ask to just sit with you, or you can trust to take care of your baby. People often want to help but are not sure how to navigate those first days and weeks of new parenting. If you don't want people over, definitely say no. But if you'd like help or company, please ask them to come over and bring a meal on their way in and bring the garbage out when they leave! You can also find more information about support groups and our warm line on our website, perinatalsupport.org.

Perinatal Support Washington
perinatalsupport.org
Warm Line 1.888.404.7763

FIGURE 12.1 (Continued)

Therapy and Therapeutic Strategies

- What was meaningful about our work together?
- What activities, insights, or concepts would you like to hold on to?
- What strategies help you calm down when stress increases?
- What do you need to remember about being a caregiver when hard moments happen? What do you need to remember about your little one in those moments?
- How would you know when you or your little one might need to make an appointment with me or with another provider?

Medications/Herbs and Supplements

- What do you need? What does your little one need?
- What works for your body? What works for your little one?
- Who can you go to for support for yourself or your child(ren)?
- What message, if any, do you need to hear from yourself regarding medications, herbs, and supplements?

Sleep Plan

- How much sleep do you need to function? How much sleep do you need to thrive in your day-to-day life?
- Is this a moment of good enough functioning or one of thriving? What do you need to remember the difference?
- When you are in a moment of good enough functioning, what do you need to do for yourself? (Consider times when babies get sick, sleep regressions, and other moments that can cause disruption.)

Support

- What community connection do you need in a moment of stress?
- What community connection do your little ones need?
- What do you need from your support system when stress increases? What do you need for you? What do you need for your children?

Tending to My Body

- What do you need to do to be a nurturing caregiver for yourself?
- What does your body need so you can be present and nurturing for your little ones?
- How will you know when you are losing a connection to your needs?

Me Time

- How much time on your own do you need to function as a person and a caregiver? To thrive?
- What activities nourish your mind, body, and soul?
- What can you realistically do in a stressful moment to care for yourself?
- What loving and compassionate message can you tell yourself when *me time* is limited?

Household Expectations

- What do you need to protect you and your child(ren) physically and emotionally?
- What compassionate message do you need to tell yourself about running your household when stress increases?

My Support Team

- Who is on your team?
- How do you let them know when you need support?
- What do they need to know to support you as a person and a caregiver?

A section you can add to the WP is *Family Time*. This part can address quality relational time between caregivers and children. When joy, love, and nurturing are low, the well-being of a relationship is at risk. Here are some questions to guide this section:

- What is quality family time?
- How much quality family time do we need to function?
- What simple activities support love, joy, and nurturing in my family?
- Who or what can help me remember family time?

Highs and lows are part of the human experience. Periods of low do not necessarily mean that people need to come back into counseling. It does mean that they need to prioritize physical and emotional wellness. Wellness during distress is a difficult task. The WP can support realistic action as people notice stress increasing. The preparation during termination can support the client in holding on to the work you did together (Vasquez et al., 2008).

SUMMARY

Like life, therapy moves through cycles. The therapeutic journey can terminate or pause depending on the circumstances of the family, the therapist, or the relationship. Discussion about the end stage of counseling must happen throughout treatment life as part of informed consent and collaboration. When therapy is or might be time-limited, therapists need to partner with clients to work at the pace of the allotted time. Therapists can explore with clients how to make meaning as sessions end. Although rituals and activities can be meaning-ful, the relationship and our attunement to clients are the agents of change. Emotional lows are a reality of the cycles of life. A WP can be a helpful tool to support planning for moments of distress when the client is no longer in session.

REFERENCES

Perinatal Support Washington (n.d.) Wellness plan. https://perinatalsupport.org/perinatal-trainings/

Tenets Initiative (2018). Diversity-informed tenets for work with infants, children & families/Principios informados en la diversidad para trabajar con bebés, niños, niñas y familias. Irving Harris Foundation. https://diversityinformedtenets.org/download-the-tenets/

Vasquez, M. J. T., Bingham, R. P., & Barnett, J. E. (2008). Psychotherapy termina-tion: Clinical and ethical responsibilities. *Journal of Clinical Psychology, 64*(5), 653–665. https://doi.org/10.1002/jclp.20478

Closing Letter to Readers

Dear Reader,

Thank you for embarking on this journey with me. I've felt your presence with me in spirit in each chapter. I hope the words in this text have supported your work and created space for reflecting deeper on your way of being with yourself and with others. As you consider expanding your perspective in serving perinatal caregivers and their little ones, please remember to hold yourself in mind with gentleness. We can recognize the areas for growth while being compassionate with ourselves in the process. We can contain both parts. However, as we tend to be our biggest critic, we might need reminders that kindness and compassion are part of the journey.

> When we choose to take a stand against oppression
> May the light of the morning sun illuminate our lives
> May we choose to move towards the light
> May we embrace the shadow
> May we be well
> May all benefit

With so much appreciation,

Meyleen

DOI: 10.4324/9781003286394-18

Appendix

Cultural Humility in Perinatal Social Work: A Toolkit for Professionals

THE TOOLKIT

This toolkit was developed as the deliverable from a qualitative action research study. The study aimed to explore how perinatal social workers can apply cultural humility.

Brief Background on the Study

Three stakeholder groups participated in this study and provided insight into how perinatal social workers can apply cultural humility. These stakeholder groups were perinatal social workers, professionals who train perinatal social workers, and social work educators.

The National Center for Health Statistics (2021) reported 3,605,201 provisional births in 2020. Considering that one in five birthing individuals may face pregnancy and postpartum complications, these numbers suggest that over 721,040 birthing people, families, and individuals may require treatment annually (CDC, n.d.). Over 50% of all individuals experiencing perinatal mental health complications do not receive proper screening or treatment (Iturralde et al., 2021).

Who Can Use this toolkit?

The information presented aims to support organizations and the perinatal social work community in determining best practices for integrating cultural humility in their work with clients. Integrating cultural humility may improve the quality of care for perinatal individuals with diverse, intersectional identities. There is limited research on how perinatal social workers can apply cultural humility in perinatal settings.

This toolkit includes information on perinatal mental health, ethics, foundational social work practices, and ways to address current challenges in applying cultural humility.

THE RESEARCH: EXECUTIVE SUMMARY

Research Purpose. This research project collected data on how social workers serving the perinatal population apply the concept of cultural humility. The study aimed to answer the research question, "How can perinatal social workers apply cultural humility?" When social workers practice from a cultural humility framework, they can increase access to care and support positive outcomes for diverse perinatal populations.

Theoretical Foundations. As social workers become aware of historical oppression, privilege, and their social locations, they understand barriers affecting marginalized communities and equalize power dynamics in the provider-client relationship. Birthing people seeking perinatal services are constantly exposed to Eurocentric, discriminatory, and oppressive treatment as they navigate the mental health system. This study's theoretical framework is anti-oppressive theory. This theory focuses on dismantling oppressive systems that harm communities.

Methodology. This qualitative action research intended to identify ways to support perinatal social workers applying cultural humility. The study utilized a generic inquiry design. Three stakeholder groups participated in semi-structured interviews: perinatal social workers, professionals who train perinatal social workers, and social work educators who teach cultural humility. The research uses purposive and snowball sampling techniques. The data was analyzed using a reflexive thematic approach. The flexible orientation of this type of analysis allowed the researcher to apply anti-oppressive theory to develop codes and themes.

Findings. The analysis revealed four themes: (a) deciding to move beyond cultural competence, (b) applying an anti-oppressive lens, (c) integrating foundational social work skills, and (d) addressing training challenges. The findings revealed that cultural humility is a complex practice beyond cultural competence, requiring an active engagement in understanding systems of oppression and biases. The results showed that social workers could integrate social work skills to reduce harm to marginalized populations when social workers are reflective. The findings also showed different barriers social workers face in learning cultural humility.

Recommendations. The recommendations include strategies for perinatal social workers and systems supporting perinatal populations. Social work trainers must represent diverse backgrounds and support providers in reflection to address internalized oppression. Systems have a responsibility to ensure that training is equitable. They also must provide training that is financially accessible and that fits within the high demands of the field.

PERINATAL MENTAL HEALTH: BACKGROUND

What is Perinatal Mental Health?

Perinatal mood and anxiety disorders like postpartum depression are the most common complication of childbirth (Parade et al., 2018). In the United States, approximately 20% of all birthing individuals experience a mood or anxiety disorder up to one year after the baby is born. Symptoms can significantly worsen when individuals experiencing perinatal mental health complications do not receive evaluation and treatment.

> Without treatment, mental health complications risk worsening, increasing the likelihood of adverse outcomes for the caregiver and infant
>
> (Taylor et al., 2019; Parade et al., 2018)

STRUCTURAL BARRIERS

These rates increase depending on the intersection of an individual's marginalized identities. During the perinatal period, individuals seeking social work services represent multiple backgrounds, experiences, and historically marginalized identities (Cooper Owens & Fett, 2019). Birthing individuals of color experience these complications at rates twice as high as their white counterparts, with conditions often going unnoticed and untreated (Keefe et al., 2016). Although changes in screening recommendations and state laws increase the early diagnosis and treatment of perinatal mental health complications, individuals with marginalized identities face significant structural barriers to care (Bubar et al., 2016).

These numbers highlight a need for adequately trained, culturally humble providers to support diverse communities.

Although academic programs, licensure bodies, and professional organizations mandate cultural competency training, clients continue to experience harm when accessing services.

PERINATAL SOCIAL WORKERS

The Role of the Perinatal Social Worker

Perinatal social workers support individuals, families, and communities through pregnancy and the first year postpartum (NAPSW, 2016). They work in various settings, including hospitals, community health, and private practice. The role of the social worker varies depending on their work setting. Some perinatal social workers might provide direct clinical interventions, discharge planning, and case management services supporting the changes and complications that the client might be experiencing.

> The perinatal period (pre-conception through a baby's first year of life) can be complicated by such factors as medically high risk pregnancies, fetal diagnosis, premature/sick newborns, drug use by the pregnant woman and/or her family, familial conflict, legal concerns, parents who have cognitive, behavioral and/or mental health needs, ambivalence about the pregnancy, and poverty. Even healthy pregnancies with optimal psychosocial conditions can be affected by anxiety and uncertainty as individuals make the transition to parenthood
>
> (National Association for Perinatal Social Workers, 2016, para. 3)

The Code of Ethics

Social workers are uniquely positioned to support communities experiencing different types of oppression as they are called to advance social justice (NASW, 2021).

Social justice, dignity and worth of the person, and competent practice are core values outlined in the NASW Code of Ethics (20). As mental health practitioners, social workers are responsible for filtering all clinical interventions through the lens of the client's culture and needs. Perinatal social workers must remain aware of the complexities an individual might experience, as a lack of proper care might negatively impact the individual, their family, and their children (Goodman, 2019).

Most clients receiving services through non-profit organizations are racial and ethnic minorities, who then receive service from professionals from dominant groups (Rosen et al., 2017). In 2020, the Council on Social Work Education (CSWE) reported that over 66% of all new social workers were White. This statistic suggests that dominant groups remain the largest service provider population and highlights the need for awareness of implicit biases and systemic barriers.

CULTURAL HUMILITY IN PERINATAL SOCIAL WORK

What is Cultural Humility?

Tervalon and Murray-Garcia conceptualized cultural humility in 1998 and defined it as "a process that requires humility as individuals to continuously engage in self-reflection and self-critique as lifelong learners and reflective practitioners" (p. 118)

Cultural humility is an approach to self-awareness and critique, preparing professionals to address power imbalances and intersecting identities that clients may experience (Sloane et al., 2018).

> It is a process that requires humility as individuals to continuously engage in self-reflection and self-critique as lifelong learners and reflective practitioners
>
> (Tervalon & Murray-Garcia, 1998, p. 118)

Power Dynamics

Examining power dynamics and intersectionality are critical parts of culturally aware and reflective practice (Lusk et al., 2017). However, many professionals are not fully competent in working with diverse and marginalized populations. When well-meaning providers fail to explore and critically self-reflect on their beliefs, values, and experiences, they inadvertently place their clients at risk of further oppression. A lack of adequate training in cultural humility leaves perinatal social workers without the skills to provide competent services to diverse populations (Hook et al., 2016). Professionals who do not practice from a critically aware framework risk further marginalizing historically oppressed groups (Rosen et al., 2017; Sloane et al., 2018).

Regarding training and competency, social workers must practice beyond the idea of "best practice" to engage in critical reflection and shifting biases.

When social workers identify and provide services early, we can prevent long-term adverse consequences for parents and children. The key to creating long-term changes rests on properly supporting clinicians.

The Life-Long Journey of the Culturally Humble Perinatal Social Worker

Deciding to move beyond cultural competency

A move beyond cultural competence calls for social workers to engage in a continuous and active process of self-examination and critique. Intentionality and action are critical for centering the client as the cultural expert.

Integrating Foundational Social Work Skills

The Code of Ethics is central to social work practice. Key features to keep active in a cultural humility practice are client self-determination, prioritizing clients' cultural needs, and practicing at the micro/mezzo/macro levels. The latter reflects a need to think beyond 1:1 client care.

Applying an anti-oppressive lens

This journey involves intentional engagement in learning about systems of oppression, recognizing biases, being aware of our social location, and being mindful of ethnocentrism. When we engage in this lens, we can support removing barriers that create harm. An intersectional lens is critical to competent client care.

Addressing Training Challenges

Training is vital to developing skills as social workers. Unfortunately, challenges exist to supporting social workers' education growth. These challenges are needing to learn from diverse sources, having an opportunity to practice new skills with support, and accessing training that meets social workers' busy lifestyles and financial needs.

Although simple sounding, cultural humility is a complex practice that requires continuous commitment and practice.

Making a Decision towards Cultural Humility

MOVING BEYOND COMPETENCE

Recommendations:

- It is recommended for training and supervision to openly discuss cultural humility as a continuous and active journey that entails self-reflection so that the social workers center their clients as cultural experts.
  - o Providers can meet this goal by providing specific reflection questions, tools, and action steps that social workers can explore to increase humility.
  - o These practices can be implemented at graduate and post-graduate levels, supporting current and future social workers.
- Another recommendation is for social workers to integrate self-reflection into everyday practice, such as in team meetings and before/after client sessions.

Applying an Anti-Oppressive Lens

THE INTERNAL WORK

Recommendations:

- Social work training can include sections discussing the history of structural racism and systemic oppression that different marginalized groups experience.
  - o These sections must be connected with outcomes so that social workers increase critical knowledge of how systemic barriers affect populations.
- A second recommendation is for training programs to provide reflective spaces where in-training and current social workers can increase their awareness of biases, social location, and ethnocentrism.
  - o Social workers can also benefit from ensuring these topics are discussed in team meetings and explored when deciding on interventions.
  - o It is also recommended that systems consider an intersectional lens to client care.
    - For example, this recommendation might require systems to develop intake assessments that ask about clients' identities in a trauma-informed way.

Integrating Foundational Social Work Skills

BACK TO BASICS

Recommendations:

- It is recommended for perinatal social worker training to encourage discussions on how organizational policies and interventions align with the NASW Code of Ethics.
- It is also recommended that perinatal social workers incorporate self-determination discussions with clients and revisit those conversations multiple times throughout service.

Addressing Training Challenges

SUPPORTING LEARNING & GROWTH

Recommendations:

- It is recommended that social workers engage in critically reflective supervision/consultation to explore their implementation of cultural humility.
- It is recommended for perinatal social workers to engage in training led by members of historically marginalized communities.
- It is also recommended that perinatal social workers engage in training that centers on decolonized and Indigenous practices.
- It is recommended that systems provide accessible training to social workers working in their communities.
  - o Systems must actively increase the visibility of diverse trainers and equitable access to this training.

RESOURCES

This section provides recommended resources for implementing cultural humility in perinatal social work.

Books

- Dunbar-Ortiz, R. (2015). *An Indigenous People's history of the United States*. Beacon Press. Kendi, I. X. (2016). *Stamped from the beginning: The definitive history of racist ideas in America*. Nation Books.

- Kendi, I. X. (2019). *How to be an anti-racist*. One World.
- Oluo, I. (2018). *So you want to talk about race*. Hatchette Press.
- Oparah, J. C., Arega, H., Hudson, D., Jones, L., & Oseguera, T. (2018). *Battling over birth: Black women and the maternal health care crisis*. Praeclarus Press.
- Piepzna-Samarasinha, L. L. (2018). *Care work: Dreaming disability justice*. Arsenal Pulp Press.
- Ross, L. J., R. L., Derkas, E., Peoples, W., & Bridgewater-Toure, P. (2017). *Radical reproductive justice: Foundations, theory, practice, critique*. Feminist Press.
- Sanders, R. (1992). *Lost tribes and promised lands: The origins of American racism*. HarperPerennial.
- Singh, A. (2019). *The racial healing handbook: Practical activities to help you challenge privilege, confront systemic racism, and engage in collective healing*. New Harbinger.

Podcast & Video

- Birth Bruja. https://www.birthbruja.com/birth-bruja-podcast.html
- Code Switch. https://www.npr.org/podcasts/510312/codeswitch
- NASW Town Hall Series on Racial Equity: Undoing Racism. https://www.youtube.com/watch?v=pkM2Y02MzQMNATAL
- https://www.natalstories.com/listen

Online Sources

- Black Lives Matter. https://blacklivesmatter.com/
- Black Mamas Matter. https://blackmamasmatter.org/
- Council on Social Work Education: Center for and Social & Economic Justice. https://www.cswe.org/Centers-Initiatives/Centers/Center-for-Diversity
- Facing History and Ourselves. https://www.facinghistory.org/
- Institute for Research and Education on Human Rights. https://www.irehr.org/
- Indigenous Social Welfare: Decolonizing Social Work. https://guides.lib.berkeley.edu/IndigenousSocialWelfare
- International Federation of Social Workers. https://www.ifsw.org/
- Human Rights Watch. https://www.hrw.org/
- Nalgona Positivoty Pride. https://www.nalgonapositivitypride.com/
- National Association of Social Workers. https://www.socialworkers.org/
- National Association of Perinatal Social Workers. https://www.napsw.org/

- National Birth Equity Collaborative. https://birthequity.org/
- Perinatal Mental Health Alliance for People of Color. https://pmhapoc.org/
- Southern Poverty Law Center. https://www.splcenter.org/
- World Association for Transgender Health. https://www.wpath.org/

Advanced Education

- Black Maternal Mental Health Summit. https://www.bmhsummit.com
- Maternal Mental Health Now: Intersectionality and Perinatal Mental Health. https://www.maternalmentalhealthnow.org/intersectionality-and-perinatal-mental-health/
- Multicultural Maternal Mental Health Conference. https://www.soysom.com/the-conference

Recommendation on Supervision/Consultation for Perinatal Social Workers

- Seek to engage in supervision/consultation with providers experienced in anti-racism and anti-oppressive practice and are members of historically marginalized communities.

REFERENCES

Bubar, R., Cespedes, K., & Bundy-Fazioli, K. (2016). Intersectionality and social work: Omissions of race, class, and sexuality in graduate school education. *Journal of Social Work Education*, *52*(3), 283–296. https://doi.org/10.1080/10437797.2016.1174636

Centers for Disease Control and Prevention. (n.d.). Depression among women. https://www.cdc.gov/reproductivehealth/depression/index.htm

Cooper Owens, D., & Fett, S. M. (2019). Black maternal and infant health: Historical legacies of slavery. *American Journal of Public Health*, *109*(10). 1342–1345.

Council on Social Work Education. (2020). The social work profession: Findings from three years of surveys of new social workers. https://cswe.org/CSWE/media/Workforce-Study/The-Social-Work-Profession-Findings-from-Three-Years-of-Surveys-of-New-Social-Workers-Dec-2020.pdf

Goodman J. H. (2019). Perinatal depression and infant mental health. *Archives of psychiatric nursing*, *33*(3), 217–224. https://doi.org/10.1016/j.apnu.2019.01.010

Hook, J. N., Farrell, J. E., Davis, D. E., DeBlaere, C., Van Tongeren, D. R., & Utsey, S. O. (2016). Cultural humility and racial microaggressions in counseling. *Journal of Counseling Psychology*, *63*(3), 269–277. https://doi.org/10.1037/cou0000114

Iturralde, E., Hsiao, C.A., Nkemere, L., Kubo, A., Sterling S. A., Flanagan, T., Avalos, L. A. (2021). Engagement in perinatal depression treatment: A qualitative study of barriers across and within racial/ethnic groups. *BMC Pregnancy Childbirth*, *21*(512), 1–11. https://doi.org/10.1186/s12884-021-03969-1

Keefe, R.H., Brownstein-Evans, C. & Rouland Polmanteer, R.S. (2016). Having our say African-American and Latina mothers provide recommendations to health and mental health providers working with new mothers living with postpartum depression. *Social Work in Mental Health*, *14*(5), 497–508. https://doi.org/10.1080/15332985.2016.1140699

National Association for Social Workers. (2021). The NASW Code of Ethics. https://www.socialworkers.org/About/Ethics/Code-of-Ethics/Code-of-Ethics-English

National Association of Perinatal Social Workers. (2016). What is a perinatal social worker? https://www.napsw.org/what-is-a-perinatal-social-worker

National Center for Health Statistics. (2021). Births: Provisional data for 2020. *Vital Statistics Rapid Release*, *12*, 1–11. https://www.cdc.gov/nchs/data/vsrr/vsrr012-508.pdf

Parade, S. H., Armstrong, L. M., Dickstein, S., & Seifer, R. (2018). Family context moderates the association of maternal postpartum depression and stability of infant temperament. *Child Development*, *89*(6), 2118–2135. https://doi.org/10.1111/cdev.12895

Rosen, D., McCall, J., & Goodkind, S. (2017). Teaching critical self-reflection through the lens of cultural humility: An assignment in a social work diversity course. *Social Work Education*, *36*(3), 289–298. https://doi.org/10.1080/02615479.2017.1287260

Sloane, H. M., David, K., Davies, J., Stamper, D., & Woodward, S. (2018). Cultural history analysis and professional humility: Historical context and social work practice. *Social Work Education*, *37*(8), 1015–1027. https://doi.org/10.1080/02615479.2018.1490710

Tervalon, M., & Murray-Garcia, J. (1998). Cultural humility versus cultural competence: A critical distinction in defining physician training outcomes in multicultural education. *Journal of Health Care for the Poor and Underserved*, *9*(2), 117–125. https://doi.org/10.1353/hpu.2010.0233

Index

Note: Locators in *italic* indicate figures, in **bold** tables and in ***bold italic*** boxes.

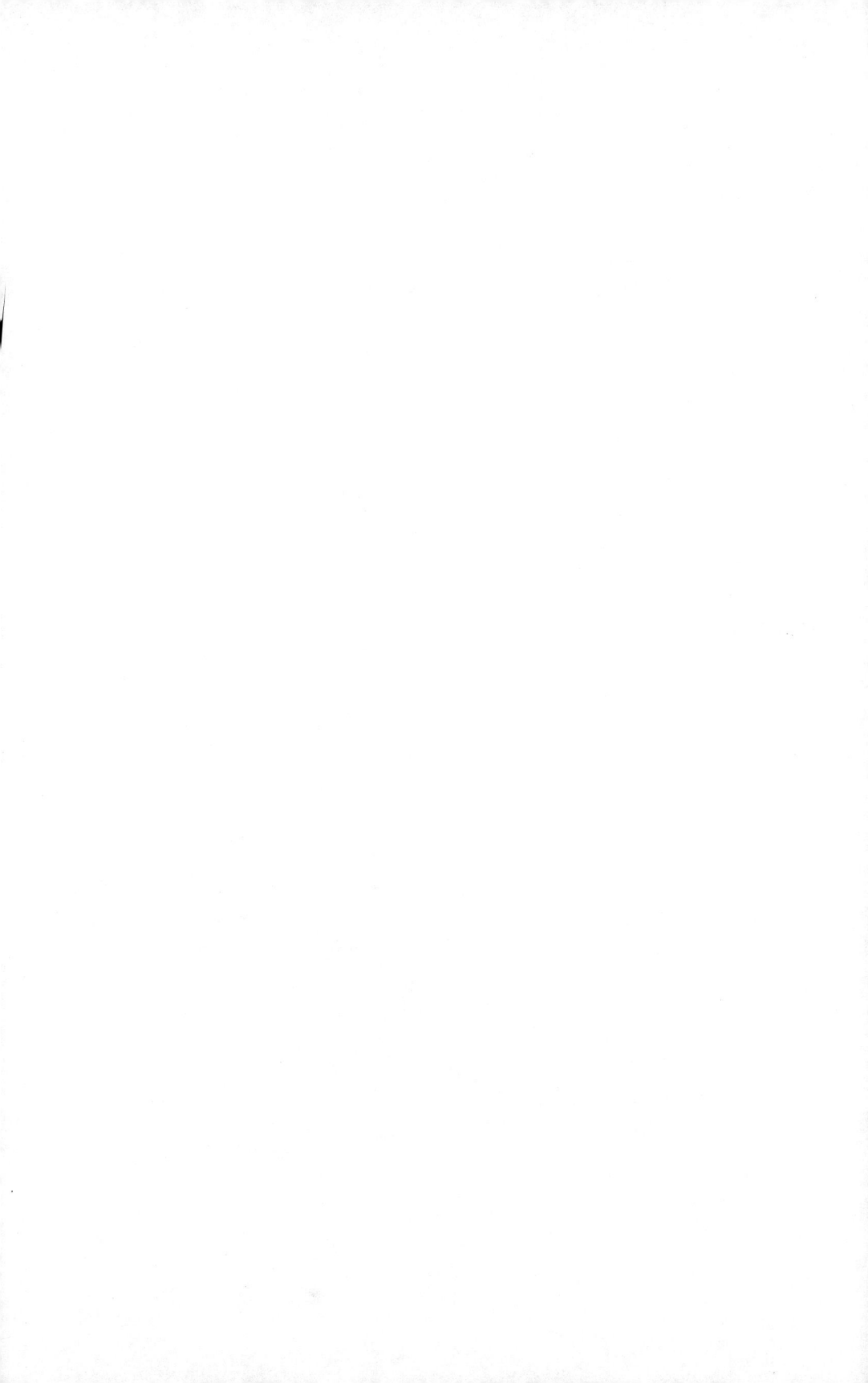